# The Best Guide to Alternative Medicine

### Paul Froemming, M.A.

*Additional material by Rick Benzel*
*Series Editor Richard F. X. O'Connor*
*Illustrations by Cathy Pavia*

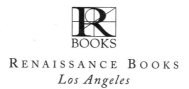

RENAISSANCE BOOKS
*Los Angeles*

*To Lisa and Michael Froemming, who illumine my life.*
*To my alma mater, the University of California at Los Angeles.*
*To my mentors in the natural and health sciences.*

Library of Congress Cataloging-in-Publication Data

Froemming, Paul.
    The best guide to alternative medicine / Paul Froemming.
        p. cm.
    Includes bibliographical references and index.
    ISBN 1-58063-017-0 (alk. paper)
    1. Alternative medicine. I. Title.
R733.F785 1998
615.5—dc21                               98-7120
                                            CIP

10 9 8 7 6 5 4 3 2 1

*Design by Lisa-Theresa Lenthall*

Distributed by St. Martin's Press
Manufactured in the United States of America
First Edition

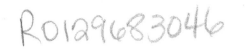
## Note to Reader

While this book contains descriptions and examples of alternative ways of dealing with health problems, they are intended to explain the various alternative traditions, not prescribe specific courses of health care action. Nothing in this book should be considered as medical advice for dealing with a given problem.

Please consult your physician if you have any questions or concerns. This book should not be regarded as a substitute for professional medical treatment. While every care has been taken to ensure the accuracy of the content, the author and the publishers cannot accept legal responsibility for any problem arising out of the use of, or experimentation with, the methods described.

In addition, it is important to note that some herbs mentioned herein may not be available in the United States, as they currently have not received approval from the Food and Drug Administration. Furthermore, herbs and nutritional supplements like vitamins can be toxic in their interaction. Consult authorities and practitioners on the subject before creating your own health modalities.

# Contents

## *Foreword*

Medicine, as we know it today, stands at an important crossroads. Around the world there are physicians, like myself, who are making use of a new resource to help their patients to recover, and to maintain, optimum health. The name of this resource is *integrative medicine,* an innovative clinical approach that combines Western technological medicine with the most powerful proven techniques from Eastern medicine. Western medicine is best known, here in the western hemisphere, as "conventional" medicine, while Eastern and other natural traditions have been called "alternative" approaches to healing. Integrative medicine seeks to combine the best ideas and practices of conventional and alternative medicine. It neither rejects conventional medicine nor embraces alternative medicine uncritically.

To take advantage of this new resource for health and healing, we; whether we be physicians, patients, health seekers, or members of other health professions, need to understand what alternative medicine is, and what it can do for us. That is where this new book, *The Best Guide to Alternative Medicine,* can help. It is organized as a true guide, allowing the reader to quickly find the alternative health information they may need at the moment.

In Part 1, The Keys to Vitality and Balance, the actual foundation for health is laid, with a practical look at food, water, breathing, exercise, and nutrition as seen from the perspective of natural healing. Throughout the book, the great healing traditions of Ayurvedic medicine, traditional Chinese medicine, naturopathy, herbal medicine, and other therapies can be seen at work.

In Part 2, The Mind/Body Connection, the effects of the mind on stress, the immune system, and brain chemistry can be found. It is now known that the mind has a powerful effect on whether we will be sick or well. Through techniques such as meditation and visualization, described in the book, readers can reduce stress and assist in their own healing process. My own practice in treating patients with symptoms of memory loss or Alzheimer's disease has convinced me that much can be done through the alternative methods of nutrition, including supplementation, stress management, and mind/body exercises, to prevent these problems. In the research for my book, *Brain Longevity,* I found that age-associated memory impairment is virtually pandemic among people of approximately age fifty, the "baby boomer" generation. Alzheimer's disease is also commonly considered inevitable for a great many people. Today, Alzheimer's strikes *up to 50 percent of all people who live to age eighty-five.* Because of this high incidence, Alzheimer's is the third-highest cause of death by disease in America, after cardiovascular disease and cancer. When baby boomers went to their local doctors for help, they'd been told that no medical protocol existed for arresting or preventing Alzheimer's disease, or for treating age-associated memory impairment. In general, the medical profession takes a lamentably passive approach to cognitive decline. According to long-standing conventional wisdom, *nothing* can stop Alzheimer's, or relieve age-associated memory impairment. But I don't accept the inescapableness of Alzheimer's, or of age-associated memory impairment. I believe that Alzheimer's disease can be delayed and prevented. I believe that age-associated memory impairment can be eradicated. I believe that people in their forties, fifties, and sixties—and beyond—can retain not only perfect memory, but can have "youthful minds," characterized by the dynamic brain power, learning ability, creativity, and emotional zest usually found only in young people. These beliefs of mine—now shared by other cutting-edge researchers and clinicians—have been considered absolutely revolutionary, but I'm positive they're true, for one central reason: the clinical results I have achieved. I have done this by applying a program that I believe is at the forefront of anti-aging medicine—a clinical approach that combines conventional medicine with alternative medicine. This book introduces the alternative methods of brain power simply and accurately, and directs the reader to the resources they will need for further study.

In Part 3, Prevention and Longevity, the miraculous immune system is described, along with ways it can best be nurtured for enhanced longevity and disease prevention. The right foods and natural methods are shown for an anticancer and heart-healthy lifestyle. Part 4 is all about healing, with 25 of the leading alternative therapies, from acupuncture to yoga, described, along with their best uses and the research that backs them up. Finally, there is a section on natural remedies for some 25 common health problems.

For the benefits of integrative medicine to work for us—as I have seen it work in my own clinical practice—we in the West need to have a new understanding and appreciation for the benefits of alternative medicine. That is what *The Best Guide to Alternative Medicine* can give us. As a bio-medical communicator in both natural healing and conventional medicine, Paul Froemming is well qualified to be your guide on a fascinating world tour of the best in alternative medicine. I wish you an interesting and successful journey.

*Dharma Singh Khalsa, M.D.*
*President/Medical Director*
*Alzheimer's Prevention Foundation, Tucson, Arizona*

## *Preface*

A book about alternative medicine is by nature a book about prevention—the prevention of health problems before they begin—for this is where this great healing tradition can have the most profound effect on our lives. By learning to live a prevention lifestyle we can enhance vitality, strength, and immunity in ways that build up the whole person—body, mind, and spirit—and strengthen our natural ability to be well. The journey to achieve these goals can often be as pleasant as the benefits themselves. Many health seekers have discovered that natural ways can be the best. For example, creating your own juices from fresh fruits and vegetables produces some of the most delicious drinks in the world. Think of fresh tomatoes with celery, or a blend of apples with lemons. That these juices are also nutrient dense, and loaded with fresh enzymes that go to work for you within minutes after juicing and drinking, is an added bonus. It is one of the alternative methods you will find in this book, called "Juice Therapy."

The spirit behind much of alternative medicine is "Resistance, Repair, and Recovery." So, if you need to recover, alternative medicine can also help in many natural ways. These ways may help you manage stress with meditation. Or they can help you recover from a cold with herbal remedies such as garlic root, boneset, and catnip, which act as antibiotics and immune system stimulants. Or, in the therapy known as mind/body medicine, they may speed your recovery from a serious disease through exercises in visualization and imagery. In my own research for writing this book I have found that western trained medical doctors are often the most enthusiastic and eloquent voices on the benefits of alternative medicine. Among those I have met with and learned from on my journey are Carl Simonton, M.D., a radiation oncologist who now practices mind/body medicine and healing visualization; Deepak Chopra, M.D., who taught me the role of spirituality in healing; and Dharma Singh Khalsa, M.D., who has made exciting breakthroughs in the area of mind, memory, and brain longevity.

In addition to prevention and recovery, alternative ways are life enhancers, as you will find in the exercise, breathing, and food therapy chapters of this book. Finally, alternative medicine is a global adventure, bringing the wisdom of Ayurvedic medicine from India, and traditional Chinese medicine into our homes, along with European and North American herbalism and naturopathy, to name but a few stops along the way. I hope you enjoy using this guide as much as I enjoyed bringing it to you.

*Paul Froemming, M.A.*
*Santa Barbara, California*

# *Acknowledgments*

The author owes a debt of gratitude to the many researchers and practitioners of the health sciences who have contributed to our knowledge of how to achieve and maintain optimum health. Their successful breakthroughs made this book possible. For sharing their wisdom and their spirit with me, I want to personally thank Deepak Chopra, M.D., Dharma Singh Khalsa, M.D., Carl Simonton, M.D., Karla Freeman, L.C.S.W., Rick Benzel, Jean Marie Stine, J. Robert Hatherill, Ph.D., Jack Rutten, M.D., and many others; and for his guidance and enthusiasm, my editor, Richard F. X. O'Connor.

# Introduction: What's Alternative about Alternative Medicine?

*T*he Western form of health care—such as that practiced in the United States, Canada, and much of Europe—often seems to be the best and the most effective medical system in the world. We have easy access to highly trained and skilled doctors, to an astonishing array of medicines that combat increasing numbers of diseases, and to sophisticated medical equipment and research facilities. Through experience, we have also learned to have hope from the constant stream of new discoveries and medical technologies that, little by little, will soon defeat the diseases we cannot currently cure.

However, over the last decades, there have been increasing voices, among both patients and health care practitioners, many asking pointed questions about Western medical practices. Among them:

- Why does conventional medicine need to be so expensive?

- Why do modern drugs have so many negative side effects?

- Why can't certain diseases be prevented and save us from bearing the pain and expense?

- Why do drugs and surgery seem to be required so often?

- Why can't doctors help us learn to be healthier and live longer, so we don't get sick in the first place?

One result of this questioning has been an opening up to other types of medicine. More and more people have been learning about and trying some of the dozens of other, distinctly different healing practices and techniques used with great success by other cultures. Many of these healing systems extend back thousands of years, and their age-old wisdom is increasingly recognized and respected among Western medical practitioners.

This book will take you on a tour of the world's various alternative healing traditions. Over the last few years, as they have gained more currency in the West, they have become referred to collectively as *alternative medicine*. Of course, they are only alternative to Westerners. Each tradition is very much mainstream in the cultures where they originated. The West considers them alternative only because they do not fall into the domain of our conventional medical system.

This book will explore a number of these traditions, present their basic principles, and offer step-by-step guidance in how you can reap their health benefits in your own life. (Omitted are several controversial diagnostic practices which are part of the ever-growing alternative medical tradition but which are unproven and may lead to misdiagnosis.)

### ALTERNATIVE MEDICAL TRADITIONS

*Acupressure*

*Acupuncture*

*Aromatherapy*

*Ayurvedic medicine*

*Chiropractic*

*Herbal therapy*

*Homeopathy*

*Massage therapy and bodywork*

*Naturopathy*

*North American folk medicine*

*Osteopathy*

*Traditional Chinese medicine*

*Yoga*

## *Alternative vs. Conventional Medicine*

What exactly makes alternative healing systems or treatments different from conventional Western medicine? Are we talking here about only minor differences in treatment style, use of drugs, or cost?

Actually, there are significant philosophical and practical differences between conventional Western medicine and nearly all alternative medical systems. The two views diverge on four fundamental issues in health care:

- What defines health?

- What causes illness?

- How does healing occur?

- Who performs healing?

These four issues overlap extensively, but for purposes of discussion, we will discuss them one at a time.

### What Defines Health?

In general, Western medicine views health as the absence of disease. In contrast, most alternative medical traditions consider health to be a positive state of well-being produced by abundant vitality. Because Western medicine focuses on disease, it generally thinks of and attempts to cure illness in the physical body—studying and treating muscles, bones, organs, tissues, cells, even molecules. Little attention has been paid to the role our psychological well-being, attitudes, beliefs, and spirit play in fostering or disrupting health.

In contrast, nearly all alternative healing traditions define wellness as an explicit state of well-being, of normal, healthy functioning—not just the absence of disease. In many alternative medical views, this state of well-being is called vitality or vital life force. This is understood, either literally or metaphorically, as a primal energy that courses through and powers the body, the way electricity in a battery powers a car. Most alternative healing traditions also believe health is a state of being in which all the systems of body, mind, and spirit work in complete balance and harmony. Whatever throws off one system, therefore affects the others. Thus, when many alternative healing traditions evaluate a patient, they consider not just the specific systems that are affected, but the whole. As a result, they are popularly referred to as holistic medicines. *Holism* refers to the theory that the whole can be greater than the sum of its individual parts.

These two concepts, a vital well-being and mind/body balance, were once foreign to Western scientific medicine, but are deeply rooted in nearly all alternative healing traditions. For example, one major tenet of Chinese medicine, which originated nearly four thousand years ago, is that the entire body pulses with energy called *chi*. This energy runs throughout the body along an invisible network of pathways called *meridians*. In the Chinese view, chi is what creates and maintains vitality. When chi flows unencumbered through the meridians, all our organs and tissues are nourished and rejuvenated—keeping us in physical and mental balance. The uninterrupted flow of chi requires getting proper nutrition, exercising, sleeping well, and avoiding excesses of any kind, including sexual, physical, and emotional. Eating the wrong foods, sleeping too little, or living an excessive lifestyle blocks chi and throws the body out of balance. Traditional Chinese medicine holds that it is imbalance or disharmony in the mind/body that creates illness.

Ayurvedic medicine, which originated nearly five thousand years ago out of the ancient Hindu philosophical and spiritual texts called the Vedas, like Chinese medicine, is based on the existence of a primal energy, which it calls *prana*. Ayurveda postulates that, when an individual's prana flows smoothly, health is maintained. It also recognizes the importance of mind/body balance. However, in Ayurveda, it is thought that everything is comprised of five basic elements—earth, air, fire, water, and space—and that these must be balanced harmoniously if we are to experience a state of well-being. Ayurveda teaches that our lifestyle choices, including our work, eating habits, exercise patterns, beliefs, and attitudes all influence our ability to maintain that balance. If we overwork, eat the wrong types of foods for our constitution, fail to exercise, or even breathe the wrong way, we throw our constitution out of balance, which leads to ill health.

We will learn more about Chinese medicine and Ayurveda later, but for now, the important thing to remember is these two major healing traditions, like most other alternative traditions, define health more proactively than Western medicine. In their view, good health demands the maintenance of a dynamic vital energy and the balance of the mind/body. In this sense, they are much more oriented toward ensuring health by preventing disease than is Western medicine.

### What Causes Illness?

Most conventional Western medicine is based on a conflict model; the body is at war with germs, viruses, carcinogens, a poor diet, and other destructive substances from the environment. (Research on gene-based illness suggests another model, that the body is a mechanism the various parts of which may be out of alignment with one another.) Most alternative healing traditions hold that illness arises from physical and/or mental disharmony.

In part, Western medicine's emphasis on seeking the causes of illness outside the body can be traced to the discovery of bacteria by Louis Pasteur in the mid-1800s. Pasteur popularized the way for Western medicine's understanding of the germ theory of illness. Pasteur's work was continued by the discovery of viruses, which further focused Western medicine's search for the cause of illness on contagious diseases that invade our systems from outside. Medical research in the twentieth century deepened this focus, with much research centered on detecting disease-producing agents, including viruses and how they mutate and spread, along with identification of many types of poisons and toxins that cause environmental diseases. Recently, Western medicine has begun to understand the nature of genetic diseases, many of which are now believed to be caused by *teratogens,* external agents that alter fetal development.

On the other hand, Western medicine admits there is a large group of illnesses it has to classify as being of unknown causes. This includes many types of cancers and autoimmune diseases in which the body appears to attack itself. However, even in these cases, Western medical researchers often have a predilection for seeking the cause in outside agents. It is only in the last few decades that Western medicine has come to understand just how important a role our mental condition can play in promoting or retarding many diseases. The past twenty years have brought greater recognition to the influence of stress and diet in heart disease and certain types of cancers.

In contrast, most alternative healing systems look within the body for the causes of illness. They believe sickness begins with an imbalance in the mind/body system, and these imbalances can be caused by poor eating habits, lack of exercise, exhaustion, sexual excess, exposure to environmental extremes such as heat or cold, and other destructive factors. Most alternative traditions also teach that strong emotions like sadness, anger, jealousy, rage, fear, grief, even a lack of inner peace or spiritual devotion, can throw off this balance and contribute to a loss of mental and physical equilibrium.

Depending on the specific alternative tradition, these imbalances in the mind/body system are seen as leading to disease in a variety of ways. In Chinese medicine, the imbalance caused by personal excesses or even by a negative emotional state leads to worsening conditions.

- The body's vital energy becomes blocked; so its vital flow is weakened throughout or in various parts of the body.

- Deprived of this vital energy, the organs in the body begin to function poorly, no longer providing vital nourishment and rejuvenation, causing illness.

In other alternative traditions, such as Ayurveda, it is thought that the blockage of vital energy allows toxins to build up in the body and these toxins are the cause of disease. Still other alternative traditions, like naturopathy, teach that imbalances weaken the body, allowing outside agents to attack the organs and tissues. Illness is the body's natural effort to defend itself, to fight back and rid itself of the outside agents.

Whatever their differences over specifics, alternative traditions, unlike Western medicine, agree the source of disease lies inside us—not outside.

### How Does Healing Occur?

Because Western medicine sees illness as caused by destructive agents like external viruses and germs attacking the body, it naturally focuses on fighting those with other agents, such as drugs or surgery. Because most alternative traditions see illness as caused by imbalances within the body, they naturally focus on various methods for restoring our lost equilibrium and harmony, allowing the body to repair itself.

Western medicine's focus on attacking disease has lead to an emphasis on fighting symptoms, particularly pain and inflammation, even though physicians recognize these are only stopgap measures to ease the pain until the disease dissipates on its own or additional medications are used. To relieve our pain, Western physicians have an arsenal of pain killers—from simple aspirin all the way up to specialized pain killers that work on specific receptors in the brain—their pharmacopoeia.

In contrast, most alternative medical traditions teach that the body has an inherent ability to heal and rid itself of disease. Most alternative traditions avoid pharmaceutical drugs, because many such drugs negatively affect the body's natural healing forces and immune system. The alternative tradition *homeopathy* is based on the medical strategy of administering very diluted amounts of therapeutic medications. Under homeopathy, which was developed in the 1790s by the German physician Samuel Hahnemann, very diluted remedies made from plant and mineral materials are given to patients. This practice follows the principle that "like cures like" and is based on a concept similar to vaccines. A substance which creates certain symptoms in a healthy person can also be used to counteract those same symptoms in an ill person. Homeopathic medicines are miniscule dosages of materials diluted to very small amounts in an effort to arouse the person's vital force and provoke the process of healing.

Rather than use expensive pharmaceuticals, alternative healing seeks to rebalance the mind/body system with natural plants, herbs, foods, and preparations made from them. For example, Chinese physicians utilize thousands of herbal formulas made according to specific formulas developed over thousands of years of investigation and usage. Rather than bringing in a battery of expensive equipment and subjecting patients to intrusive tests, Chinese health practitioners look for four pairs of opposite and complementary indicators that show where in the body the disharmony might be occurring:

- Is it an interior organ or bone vs. exterior skin?

- Does the disease cause hot (fever and thirst) or cold (chills and need for warmth)?

- Is the illness acute or chronic?

- Does the illness reflect a yin or yang deficiency or excess? In the Chinese worldview, yin and yang are the two opposite energies that make up the universe—and us—and illness will usually reflect either a deficiency or excess of one or the other. (The concepts of yin and yang are explained in greater detail in Part 1.)

Following this diagnosis, a Chinese health practitioner will usually prescribe a specific formula of herbs proven to strengthen the organ identified as the location of the energy blockage. Strengthening this organ helps to rebalance the body, as well as remove the excess heat or chills, and resolve any yin/yang energy deficiency or excess.

Many alternative medical traditions, such as naturopathy, also aim at rebalancing the body with various corrective therapies, including massage, hot or cold baths, and exercise. Their goal is to reinvigorate the circulatory system and stimulate the internal organs in an effort to remove the toxins that are blocking the vital energy and causing the imbalances—thus restoring the body to health and banishing illness from the body.

Western and alternative medicine also diverge in their attitude toward symptoms. In the view of alternative medicine, symptoms aren't a problem to be cured, but a critical part of the body's natural effort to fight off disease. Inflammation around a wound is now known to be part of a natural process in which the body cordons off an injured area to prevent infection from seeping into other areas. Meanwhile, the increased flow of blood to the infected area rejuvenates the wound and nourishes the skin. In consequence, alternative therapies do not try to squelch symptoms. They see them as indications that the body's natural disease fighting

*"Integrative medicine seeks to combine the best ideas and practices of conventional and alternative medicine. It neither rejects conventional medicine nor embraces alternative medicine uncritically."*

—*Dharma Singh Khalsa, M.D., a Western educated physician who successfully integrates alternative therapies in his practice* mechanisms are at work, and attempt to aid them in their natural course toward healing.

A corollary of this attitude is that most forms of alternative medicine believe that the body should be allowed to operate naturally and at its own pace, aided by natural methods that help it heal itself from within. This is why it is sometimes said that Western medicine seeks to cure illnesses, while alternative medicine seeks to heal them.

### Who Performs Healing?

In general, with Western medicine the physician plays the most important role in the healing process. In the West, we look to physicians for our healing. They are the experts, the keepers of collective medical wisdom and knowledge. They are expected to rigorously analyze our symptoms, diagnose our illness, and develop an effective plan of treatment.

*Alternative healing traditions, because of their view that both health and healing come from within, believe it is the patient who plays the most important role in healing any disease or illness.* The individual, not only the physician, must be responsible for their own wellness. Among the steps we must take to preserve our well-being are:

- Eating properly

- Getting enough sleep

- Exercising at least three days weekly

- Breathing plenty of fresh, clean air

- Avoiding physical and emotional excesses that wear down the body, mind, and spirit

An alternative physician makes a diagnosis and devises a treatment for an ill patient, just as a Western doctor does, and it is well understood between doctor and patient that the patient must make whatever lifestyle changes are required and adhere to the therapies prescribed—or healing will not occur. These changes can include modifying the diet, taking vitamin supplements or natural herbal tonics, deep breathing, and various exercises.

Over the past four decades, Western medicine has increasingly accentuated the role of specialists, doctors who focus their practice on a single health topic or area of the body, in curing illness. The growth of specialists reflects the medical community's belief that the patient's wellness depends on extremely detailed research and intervention from outside. In contrast, most alternative traditions train their practitioners to be generalists who understand the links between the various body systems and who can see the whole picture rather than just a specific set of symptoms.

Secondly, because of its foundation in science, Western medicine tends to treat health care in a processed manner. Patients can easily become charts and statistics in Western medicine, not simply because dozens of patients are seen each day, but because Western preference for scientific analysis inherently emphasizes objectivity and the collecting of data in a highly organized, complementary manner.

Third, because many alternative healing traditions teach that each individual has a specific constitution and each illness reflects a lifestyle issue unique to that person, alternative physicians focus on highly individualized care rather than statistical averages and information gathering. Whether it is traditional Chinese medicine, Ayurveda, naturopathy, homeopathy, or almost any other alternative treatment, the typical alternative physician must get to know each patient in detail to understand their unique health needs and prepare a highly individualized program based on the patient's condition, body type, dietary habits, exercise level, sexual lifestyle, vitality, and other factors.

## No One Right Medical View

As you can see, Western and alternative medicine differ considerably on these fundamental issues. The following chart summarizes these basic philosophical differences:

## DIFFERENCES IN PHILOSOPHY BETWEEN CONVENTIONAL AND ALTERNATIVE MEDICINE

| *Conventional Medicine* | *Alternative Medicine* |
|---|---|
| Health is the absence of disease. | Health is a proactive state of well-being, characterized by vitality and mind/body balance. |
| The focus is generally on the cure of the disease. (However, Western medicine has recognized the correlation between lifestyle and disease.) | Health requires the maintenance of one's vitality and balance. Prevention is thus an automatic aspect of health, evident in each lifestyle decision made on a daily basis. |
| The mind and body are generally treated separately in regard to the cause and cure of disease. | The mind and body are unified; what affects one affects the other. |
| Most disease is the result of causative agents; such as bacteria, viruses, carcinogens, cancer cells, environmental factors, stress, or outside influences. | Disease originates from within, the result of an imbalance in the mind/body system that blocks the vital energy and disrupts the normal functioning of the organs. Imbalances result from excesses in lifestyle and inner disharmonies. |
| Healing requires the use of outside agents more powerful than the disease to cure it. The primary methods of healing are through the use of drugs and other methods to attack the cause of the disease and eradicate the symptoms, or through surgery and radiation. | The body has a natural ability to heal itself. Illness must be approached from within, by restoring balance and harmony to the mind/body system. Primary treatments include diet, exercise, stress management, social support, and herbal medicines, all of which restore vitality and balance in the body. |
| The best healing is to destroy the invading agents and restore normalcy. | The best healing is slow and natural, letting the body do its own work. |
| The doctor plays the pivotal role in healing; and is the one who has the medical knowledge needed to diagnose an illness and prescribe the treatment. | The patient plays the most important role in healing. The patient must heal from within. The patient's lifestyle choices influence the progress of healing. |
| Medicine is practiced using statistics and averages, along with a thorough health history and physical examination, to determine diagnoses and treatments. | Medicine is practiced on a highly individualized basis; each person requires a diagnosis and treatment according to his or her unique constitution, body type, other mental, physical and spiritual factors, and health condition. |

A debate on philosophy and practice in various medical traditions has gone on for decades. The following lists compare the strengths and weaknesses of alternative and conventional medicine.

### Conventional medicine can:

Diagnose and treat medical and surgical emergencies and trauma.

Treat acute bacterial infections with antibiotics.

Treat infections.

Prevent many infectious diseases by immunization.

Replace damaged hips, knees, and other body parts.

Perform cosmetic and reconstructive surgery.

### Conventional medicine cannot:

Cure most chronic degenerative diseases.

Cure most forms of allergy or autoimmune disease.

Effectively manage psychosomatic illnesses.

Cure most forms of cancer.

Effectively manage many kinds of mental illness.

Diagnose and correct hormonal deficiencies.

### Alternative medicine can:

Aid in preventing, alleviating, or postponing many lifestyle diseases.

Help reduce or eliminate stress.

Remedy many conditions which are not life-threatening without harsh drugs and side effects.

Reduce pain using natural methods.

Ameliorate a patient's psychological condition during illness.

Give patients a sense of dignity in the health care process.

Improve the recovery process after surgery.

### Alternative medicine cannot:

Manage trauma as well as conventional medicine.

Diagnose and treat medical and surgical emergencies as well as conventional medicine.

Improve Western methods of surgery.

Prevent many infectious diseases by immunization.

Replace damaged hips and knees.

Treat acute bacterial infections.

## Integrative Medicine

Ultimately, the convergence of Western and alternative medical practitioners has led to a new type of medicine, called *integrative medicine* that utilizes the best elements from both practices.

Integrative medicine embraces three crucial characteristics:

- An emphasis on lifelong health and disease prevention: Practitioners of integrative medicine educate their patients about the central role they play in their own healthcare, and how their lifestyle choices regarding diet, exercise, and work habits influence the quality and length of their life.

- A willingness to consider treatments and modalities from all traditions: Treatments combine the best practices from Western and alternative therapies, with the goal of choosing and matching the correct healing therapy with the patient's individual condition and personality. Some health problems seem to respond best to Western style care, such as drugs and surgery. Other conditions are best healed with alternative remedies, such as herbal medicine, diet, exercise, or stress-reduction techniques.

- A willingness to allow for simultaneous treatment plans: seeks to heal illness with techniques drawn from several traditions that complement and support each other. For example, after an injury, Western drug treatment might be the best way to reduce the immediate danger from an infection, traditional Chinese medicine might provide the best way to help reduce pain, and Ayurveda might suggest lifestyle changes that will prevent a repetition of the problem.

The main objective in *The Best Guide to Alternative Medicine* is to give you, the reader, a choice: the choice of new ways to view your health problems through alternative health practices. A second objective is to introduce you to some of the many ways your life and longevity can benefit from alternative healing. Here, then, is the best of alternative medicine.

*"Do not seek help from a conventional doctor for a condition that conventional medicine cannot treat, and do not rely on an alternative provider for a condition that conventional medicine can manage well."*

—*Andrew Weil, M.D.,*
The Ultimate Direction:
Integrative Medicine

# *The Keys to Vitality*

# *and Balance*

In Part 1, the reader will tour the great natural healing systems of the world in search of the keys to vitality and balance. In traditional Chinese medicine and acupuncture therapy, vitality is called *chi* meaning vital energy. Ayurvedic medicine views the body as filled with energy, which it calls *prana*. Naturopaths call it the vital force of life. Homeopaths seek to influence the vital force, or energetic level of the body. While they may call vitality by different names, they all agree essentially with what the dictionary defines as "liveliness, vigor, and persistent energy, connected with and essential to life."

Each of us would be happy to manifest great vitality in our lives. The healing traditions explored in Part 1 all agree that outward vitality is, indeed, a prerequisite for a life of optimum health, resistance to disease, and longevity.

# *Vitality and Diet in Alternative Medicine*

*D*iet is perhaps the first and foremost element in the concept of vitality among alternative traditions. In traditional Chinese, Ayurvedic, and naturopathic medicines, the intuitive wisdom that "you are what you eat" has been engrained for thousands of years. These traditions did not have today's science to understand the linkage between cholesterol and heart disease, free radicals and cancer, or proteins and energy. But their practitioners clearly recognized from simple observation and experience that the healthier foods a person ate, the more vital and disease-resistant that individual was, and the more likely to live an energetic, long life.

In particular, three alternative health traditions have highly developed concepts about diet and vitality: Ayurveda, Chinese, and macrobiotic. Let's begin by examining the nutritional beliefs arising out of these traditions.

## *The Ayurvedic Approach to Food*

Ayurvedic medicine is founded on the ancient Hindu philosophical and spiritual beliefs, called the Vedas, created over five thousand years ago. The Vedas encompassed what the holy men of India received as divine wisdom in four areas of human conduct: self-knowledge, the cosmology of the universe, the path to god, and physical health. For many medical scholars, Ayurveda is considered the oldest natural healing system in the world.

As mentioned in the Introduction, Ayurveda believes the body and mind are animated with a vital energy, *prana*, which is critical to the maintenance of life. Each of us is endowed with prana, but it must be continuously guarded and replenished through our actions. One primary method of rejuvenating prana was through special breathing exercises, called *pranayama*. In the Ayurvedic tradition, air is thought to contain the vital energy. (Some of these special breathing exercises will be presented in Chapter 6.)

In addition to the concept of prana, Ayurveda also held that each person is a combination of the five primary elements of the universe—air, water, earth, fire, and space. The pattern of our combination when we are born is our individual constitution. To understand human behavior, Ayurveda organizes the possible combinations of elements into three broad categories, called *doshas:*

- *Vata* (space and air)—light and airy; governs the nervous system; indicative of an active, alert personality type;

- *Pitta* (fire and water)—flowing and fiery; governs the digestive system; indicative of an aggressive, can-do personality type;

- *Kapha* (earth and water)—slow and strong; governs the bones, muscles, and healing; indicative of a steady, tranquil personality type.

The three types—vata, pitta, and kapha—are similar in some degree to the way that Western science categorizes body types. In the West, we call them ectomorph, endomorph, and mesomorph. The difference is that Ayurveda equates psychological, emotional, and spiritual characteristics with each dosha type. The following chart shows the characteristics traditionally attributed to each type.

*"Macrobiotics does not offer a single diet for everyone, but a dietary principle that takes into account differing climatic and geographical considerations, varying ages, sexes and levels of activity, and ever-changing personal needs."*

*—Michio Kushi, a leading teacher in the macrobiotic movement*

## THE PRIMARY AYURVEDIC PERSONALITY TYPES

| *Vata* (air & space) | *Pitta* (fire & water) | *Kapha* (water & earth) |
|---|---|---|
| Qualities are dry, cold, mobile, light, changeable, subtle, rough, and quick. | Qualities are hot, sharp, light, moist, slightly oily, and fluid. | Qualities are heavy, cold, oily, sweet, steady, soft, and slow. |
| Slender and light build. | Medium physique, strong, well built; blond, light brown, or red hair; fair or reddish skin. Avoids sun and hot weather. | Physically strong with a sturdy, heavier build. Tendency to be overweight. Skin is cool, pale, smooth, sometimes oily. |
| Energy comes in bursts. Walks quickly. Like the wind, they are always moving. | Medium strength and endurance. Walks with a determined stride. | Energy is steady. |
| Excitability, changing moods. Displays bursts of emotion that are short-lived and quickly forgotten. | Becomes irritable when stressed. | Possessive, affectionate, forgiving. Slow to anger. Relaxed. |
| Enthusiasm, imagination, vivaciousness, tendency to worry. | Intense, ambitious. | Happy with the status quo. |
| Irregular hunger and digestion. Digests foods well one day and poorly the next. Tendency to be constipated. | Strong appetite. Cannot skip meals. | Eats to feel emotional comfort. |
| Quick to grasp (and to forget) new information. | Bright intellect. Precise speech. | Thinks things over a long time before reaching a decision. Slow and graceful. |
| Performs activity quickly. Loves excitement and constant change. | Takes command. Enterprising. Hates to waste time. | Easygoing personality, laid back. |
| Goes to sleep at different times every night, skips meals, and keeps irregular habits in general. Tendency toward insomnia, light sleeper. Tires easily. | | Deep sleeper. Wakes up slowly. |

Each person falls into one of the three pure doshas or may be a combination of two or more of them. This means that Ayurveda recognizes seven basic personality and body types:

| Single-dosha | Double-dosha | Tri-dosha |
|---|---|---|
| vata | vata-pitta | vata-pitta-kapha |
| pitta | pitta-kapha | |
| kapha | vata-kapha | |

### Matching Your Diet to Your Dosha

The Ayurvedic concept of a personal constitution is pivotal to its nutritional and medical philosophy. Ayurveda teaches that each person must strive to live life in accordance with his or her constitution. Living contrary to one's personality creates imbalance, which leads to the buildup of toxins in the person, a skewing of the person's primary dosha, and ultimately a loss of health. Imbalances can occur from eating a diet contrary to one's personality type, inadequate rest, exposure to toxins, stress, and excessive emotions, such as fear, envy, and greed.

Diet is thus considered a critical factor in maintaining balance, personal harmony, and health in the Ayurvedic tradition. Recommendations about diet are found in a system of food guidelines for each personality type, formulated in terms of what each person must eat to balance the fluctuations in his or her constitution each day.

One dietary guideline is known as the "six tastes," in which foods are divided into their primary tastes as follows:

- *Sweet*—sugar, milk, butter, rice, bread, pasta

- *Salty*—salt

- *Sour*—yogurt, cheese, lemon

- *Pungent*—ginger, cumin, other spicy foods

- *Bitter*—green leaf vegetables, turmeric

- *Astringent*—beans, lentils, pomegranates

*Balancing the Doshas*

In Ayurveda, the main meal of the day is intended to include all six tastes, in proportion to what each person needs to maintain his or her natural constitution. Each taste was determined to perform a balancing or aggravating function on the dosha, so that once you knew your dosha you would adjust your menu as follows:

### SIX TASTES

|  | *Tastes Which Aggravate* | *Tastes Which Balance* |
|---|---|---|
| *Vata* | Pungent, bitter, astringent | Sweet, sour, salty |
| *Pitta* | Sour, salty, pungent | Sweet, bitter, astringent |
| *Kapha* | Sweet, sour, salty | Pungent, bitter, astringent |

The second part of Ayurvedic food guidelines is called the "six qualities." These have to do with the effects that certain foods have on the body. Each quality occurs in a pair as follows:

| *Heavy vs. Light* | *Oily vs. Dry* | *Hot vs. Cold* |
|---|---|---|
| *Heavy*—Beef, cheese, wheat | *Oily*—Soybeans, milk, coconut | *Hot*—Eggs, honey, pepper |
| *Light*—Chicken, skim milk, barley | *Dry*—Lentils, honey, cabbage | *Cold*—Milk, sugar, mint |

By linking the six tastes, the six qualities, and the three doshas, each person can determine what kinds of foods will balance or aggravate each body type. For example:

- *Vata*—Balanced by sweet, sour, salty; heavy, oily, hot. Aggravated by pungent, bitter, astringent; light, dry, cold.

Hence, vatas thrive on rice, breads, pasta, yogurt, grapefruit, and salty foods.

- *Pitta*—Balanced by sweet, bitter, and astringent; heavy, dry, cold. Aggravated by sour, salty, pungent; hot, light, oily.

Hence, pittas do well on leafy greens, beans, and peas.

- *Kapha*—Balanced by pungent, bitter, astringent; light, dry, hot. Aggravated by sweet, sour, salty; heavy, oily, cold.

Hence, kaphas, who have a tendency to be overweight fare best with hot and spicy foods.

As you can see, the Ayurvedic diet is highly systemized for maintaining the health and harmony of one's personality type. Not surprisingly, the system also gives credence to food intuition. If a person had a craving for a certain taste, it was a sign their body needed that type of food to rebalance their constitution. Maintaining one's health therefore requires you to be very sensitive to what your body subtly communicates to you about its needs.

Ayurveda also uses food in its healing therapies. Because Ayurvedic medicine believes each personality type is prone to certain types of diseases, Ayurvedic doctors typically prescribe dietary changes based on which foods the patient needs to increase to balance his or her dosha, or to cut out to avoid aggravating his or her dosha. For example, it is said that vata people are more susceptible to intestinal conditions, lower back pain, arthritis, and nervous system diseases. Pitta types are more likely to have liver and bile disorders, hyperacidity, gall bladder, gastritis, inflammatory diseases, and skin disorders. Kapha types are prone to congestive conditions such as bronchitis, sinusitis, and tonsillitis. For each ailment, Ayurvedic medicine thus has a dietary prescription indicating what foods to eat and which to avoid. For instance, a person with a liver condition arising out of stress and poor eating habits needs to eat foods to restore his pitta constitution and avoid foods that aggravate his vata from the stress.

### The Relevance of Ayurvedic Nutrition Today
The Ayurvedic personality types are without doubt the earliest forerunners of the various typologies psychologists have created in

the twentieth century in an effort to better understand and categorize human behavior. Although psychologists today do not correlate personality type with diet, there is an interesting point to consider that does seem to create linkage between our culture and our diseases.

Most nutritionists complain that Western culture emphasizes sweet, salty, and sour foods. According to Ayurveda, an excess of these foods leads to physical imbalances, which may cause or aggravate stress-related diseases and chronic digestive problems. If you accept the Ayurvedic concepts, it is not surprising that Westerners seem to be much more prone to stress-related diseases and digestive problems than other cultures whose diets include much less salt and sugared foods. As William Collinge, Ph.D., author of *The American Holistic Association Complete Guide to Alternative Medicine,* writes: "Ayurveda offers some very interesting insights into why we face the diseases that are so prevalent in modern societies. Because vata governs the nervous system, it is the dosha that is most easily thrown out of balance by chronic stress. The hectic, fast-paced lifestyle that many follow in Western society thus contributes to vata imbalances on a mass scale. . . . One consequence is that this translates into dietary behavior on a mass scale, involving craving for sweet, sour, and salty tastes. These tastes accompany foods that, if consumed in inordinate quantities, bring the predictably negative health effects of excess sugar, fat, and salt intake."

Collinge goes on to point out that the Western diet also appears to be related to why we have far more people with chronic

> ## THE IMPORTANCE OF DIGESTION IN THE AYURVEDIC TRADITION
>
> *In addition to its dietary recommendations, Ayurveda also includes a strong medical view about the processes of digestion and elimination. An important corollary principle in the Ayurvedic view of diet is that digestion must be complete to eliminate toxins from the body. Ayurvedic doctors were among the first to pay great attention to a person's urine and feces as indicative of a state of well-being. In addition, how a person sweats was considered an important indication of body elimination.*
>
> *Ayurveda also teaches maxims about good habits in eating. For example, it is common in Indian culture to sit down to eat and not to talk while chewing. These habits all reflect the culture's emphasis on good digestion.*

fatigue syndrome than other cultures. He attributes chronic fatigue to a breakdown in the immune system, which according to Ayurveda results from vata imbalances.

## Traditional Chinese Philosophy and Food Therapy

Traditional Chinese philosophy also considers food a key factor in health. In the Taoist view, the quality of food, nutrients in the diet, and the efficiency by which they are digested and metabolized, determine the quality of the two fluids, or essences, that form the foundation of human life: chi (the vital energy) and blood. The traditional Chinese view of human physiology focuses on two organs, the stomach and the spleen, both involved in transforming food into chi and blood.

As a result, traditional Chinese medicine believes that a lack of proper food or an excess of food can have disastrous health results. The lack of proper nourishment leads to a deficiency of chi and blood, which cause organs to malfunction. Or an excess of food can cause stagnation in energy and blood, which lead to malfunctions in the stomach.

Taoist nutritional science also believes that improper food choices can have a negative effect on health. The Chinese believe that foods not only contain nutrients that transform into chi energy and blood, but also reflect the two bioenergetic polarities of the universe, *yin* and *yang*, present in everything. Yang foods are stimulating and warm, while yin foods are calming and

---

**CHINESE MEDICINAL SOUPS**

*Food as medicine is a time-honored concept in Chinese medicine, a practice that can be literally translated as eat medicine. One example of this practice is the medicinal soups that are prepared as special treats for the whole family. While the quantities of soup are prepared according to the number of people at the meal, the recipes for the medicinal herbs included tend to remain constant. Here is an example:*

*Chinese Yam and Chinese Wolfberry Soup*

*This soup is prepared as a meat soup using lean meat, to which is added ten to thirty grams of Chinese yam (Dioscorea batatas) and six to fifteen grams of Chinese wolfberry seeds (Lycium chinese). The healthful benefits come from the yam, which strengthens the lungs, kidneys, stomach, and spleen. Wolfberry seeds, another medicinal herb, are used in the treatment of diabetes, and are thought to be restoratives to the liver and kidneys.*

cooling. Foods must be selected to balance the yin and yang qualities of the body's organs, or the yin and yang conditions outside of the body. Consider the following food remedies:

- A person who feels depressed (yin) should take yang foods for balance.

- If the weather is yin (damp and cold), yang foods are warming and will help dry the inner organs.

- Fatty and greasy foods, alcohol, or sweets can result in a condition known as Dampness and Heat.

- Too much raw food in the diet may strain the yang aspect of the spleen and cause the condition Internal Cold Dampness, characterized by abdominal pain and weakness.

### Chinese Seasonal Foods

Another element of Chinese food therapy is eating foods according to the seasons in which they are produced. While this is now becoming popular among holistic nutritionists in the West, the Chinese have been doing this for millennia. The yang foods warmed them in the winter, and the yin foods cooled them in the summer.

Here are some examples of yin and yang foods:

| *Yang (Warming) Food* | *Yin (Cooling) Food* |
| --- | --- |
| cooked vegetables | raw vegetables |
| tomato sauce | rice |
| kidney beans, lentils | yogurt |
| potatoes | bean curd (tofu) |
| cooked fish | milk |
| garlic | curry powder |
| miso | sashimi (raw fish) |
| molasses | sugar |
| cloves | salt |

*"When essence is deficient, replenish it with food."*
—Internal Medicine Classic
*(Ancient Chinese medical book)*

*Chinese Food Therapy Today*

Albert Einstein, in his formula regarding energy and matter, stated it as $E=MC^2$. The corresponding Chinese medicine and Taoist principle is *jing hwa chi*, which means "essence transforms into energy."

---

### VITALITY AND TRADITIONAL CHINESE MEDICINE

*The Taoist tradition of health and well-being, upon which Chinese medicine is founded, recognizes three aspects of life that are called the three treasures (san bao), also known as the three marvels (san chi). All humans, the tradition teaches, are endowed with these treasures at birth, and how well they care for them will determine how well, and how long, they will live. The three treasures are:*

- *Jing—The physical body and its essential fluids are called jing, meaning essence. Essence is also translated as vitality.*

- *Chi—The vital force that empowers the body and initiates life functions is called chi, meaning energy. Energy is the vital force that moves every system of the body, both conscious and autonomic.*

- *Shen—All aspects of the mind, consciousness, and cognition are known as shen, meaning spirit. Spirit is, in the final definition, the force of creation.*

*To form the Chinese word for vitality you need to combine the characters for essence (jing) and energy (chi) to form the word jing-chi. If you were to combine the characters for essence and spirit, to form the word jing-shen, you would also be saying vitality. Vitality is manifested as mental vigor, immunity, resistance to disease, and sexual potency. The main indicator of health in the Chinese system is vitality.*

---

In literal terms, there can be no doubt the transformation of essence into energy is carried out by the foods we eat and the enzymes they contain. Enzymes are produced in the mitochondria of cells. Aside from the enzymes produced in the body, the best source of food enzymes is fresh whole foods, eaten as close as possible to their natural state. This is why the Chinese diet emphasizes many fresh, semi-raw, and slightly cooked ingredients.

In contrast, the Standard American Diet, ironically known to nutritionists by the initials SAD, is almost totally lacking in enzymes, and suffers even further from so much processing and additives in our foods. One prime example of the SAD diet is the use of hydrogenated vegetable oils, such as those found in margarine and many processed foods. Hydrogenation changes these vegetable oils into harmful trans-fats that have been linked to heart disease and cancer.

Ultimately, one might say there is much wisdom in the ancient Chinese view of food. The Chinese diet emphasizes natural food alchemy taking place inside the body, by the virtue of food enzyme activity, instead of the synthetic food alchemy that we now accept in the packaged processed goods the Western consumer has been conditioned to buy. The Chinese reliance on food as medicine, and as a primary maintainer of health, as opposed to a reliance on drugs and surgery, is one of the main practices that differentiates traditional Chinese medicine from conventional Western medicine.

## Macrobiotics and Food Therapy

Macrobiotics is both a diet and a philosophy of life. As the name implies, it takes a large (macro) view of life (biotics). Macrobiotics, in its present form was developed in Japan as a personal philosophy involving wholesome living and eating. Food is considered central to life, and the macrobiotic diet is selected very carefully. The principles of yin and yang, the theory of opposites, are the guiding decision in selecting foods for the diet. Whole grains, like brown rice, contain a balance of yin and yang, and are a staple of macrobiotic eating, comprising about half of each day's nourishment. The diet can be prepared vegetarian or non-vegetarian, but dairy products are not used. Vegetables are important, including the sea vegetables of the traditional Japanese diet, on which the macrobiotic diet is based. A basic macrobiotic principle is whole food—no waste.

According to macrobiotic teaching, three types of foods to avoid are:

- Overly concentrated foods, like red meats, cheese, and eggs.

- Overly dispersing-expanding foods like simple sugars and artificial sweeteners. These are found in soft drinks, candy, and chocolate.

- Overly congesting-congealing foods like dairy products, greasy foods, and nut butters.

Four types of food to use for health are:

- High quality vegetable-based foods.

- A variety of whole grain foods (not just the brown rice with which macrobiotics is so closely associated).

- High quality vegetable proteins. Primary sources of vegetable protein are considered to be beans, tofu, and tempeh (a soy product). If animal protein is selected, seafood is recommended as best. Seafood comes from a world of water, which is more ancient and primitive than human life and less yang than other animal foods.

- Natural sweets, like honey, rice syrup, and maple syrup should be eaten in moderation. Fruits, which are also natural sweets, are best eaten separately from a main meal. Fruits are not considered to mix well with proteins. Some fruits, like the apples in applesauce, are considered more digestible after they have been cooked.

## Chapter Recap

- Ayurvedic medicine recommends a diet based on your unique constitution, to rejuvenate it on a daily basis or rebalance it when you are ill.

- Chinese medicine recommends a diet of fresh whole foods, eaten according to what is most seasonal to maintain your vitality, blood production, and inner yin/yang organ harmony.

- The macrobiotic philosophy recommends a diet based on brown rice plus vegetables and, if meat is needed, mostly fish.

*Recommended Reading*
Chopra, Deepak, M.D. *Boundless Energy: The Complete Mind/Body Program for Overcoming Chronic Fatigue.* New York: Three Rivers Press, 1995.

# *Nourishment for Vitality—Western Style*

*U*nlike the Ayurvedic, Chinese, and macrobiotic traditions, conventional Western medicine has largely neglected looking at diet from a health and disease-prevention point of view. As for consumers, our dietary knowledge is usually based on the simplistic adage: "Eat three square meals a day," which until recently has simply meant each meal must contain a balance of proteins, carbohydrates, and fats.

The evolution of the food business in the twentieth century has also been an especially negative factor in our understanding of the relationship between food and health. As farming has increasingly moved to highly industrialized production techniques and the distribution of food has been increasingly commercialized, we have become conditioned to accept fruits and vegetables grown in fields saturated with chemical fertilizers, meats from animals nourished with synthetic feeds and hormones, and highly processed sugary and salty foods wrapped in pretty packaging.

Our culture has paid a hefty price, healthwise, for this dietary heritage. In the U.S., nearly one-third of the population is overweight because of a diet loaded with too many fats, sugars, and processed foods. Heart disease and cancer have thus become the two

*IN THIS CHAPTER:*

- *Changes in the modern Western diet*

- *Science discovers phytonutrients, plant chemicals that promote health and fight disease*

- *Whole foods as the best sources*

- *Anticancer vegetables*

- *Natural antibiotics*

- *Saturated, polyunsaturated, monounsaturated—what's the difference?*

- *Olive oil to the rescue*

- *Omega-3 fatty acids*

- *High quality protein sources*

leading causes of death in many Western countries, and most physicians blame our diet as the major factor, or a contributing factor.

Fortunately, the good news is that the past decade has ushered in many new advances in understanding the link between diet and good health. Through numerous research studies and sophisticated laboratory analysis, Western scientists have made tremendous progress in identifying the complex interactions of food nutrients in the body. The effect of this is that there is now a growing segment of what might be called alternative Western medicine that focuses on nutrition and preventive food therapy in the same way many alternative traditions have always done.

This chapter reviews the ways in which Western medicine has begun to embrace preventive nutrition.

## Eat Whole Foods

The first and most important transformation Western medicine has made is understanding that the ancient cultures were wise to eat *whole* foods. Years of scientific research have proven that deriving our nutrients from whole foods rather than through processed foods or food supplements such as vitamins, is by far the most effective way to stay healthy and prevent disease. Research shows that you are helping your own health if you eat whole foods, including whole grains, whole fruits (rather than just the juice), and whole vegetables. Nutritionists recommend that you get your fruits and vegetables from fresh and organic sources, such as a farmer's market.

### WHICH IS BETTER—THE CARROT OR THE CAPSULE?

*As an example of the difference between eating whole foods or trying to obtain nutrition from a pill, consider this example. Many manufacturers now produce capsules containing beta-carotene, the substance in carrots that converts to vitamin A in the body, which has been shown to be an antioxidant that can prevent cancer. Although these supplementary capsules are an effective and inexpensive way to add beta-carotene to your diet, they come nowhere near the potency of whole foods that contain over five hundred carotenoids. Furthermore, research has shown that at least fifty of these carotenoids, including beta-carotene, are converted to vitamin A in the body. In short, it's impossible to fool the body when it comes to deriving the right nutrition.*

*Eat from the Base of the Pyramid*

With this new recognition on the value of whole foods, the old adage of eating three square meals a day has recently been replaced with a new model of what to emphasize on a daily basis in one's diet. This new model modifies the old idea that there are three primary food groups (proteins, carbohydrates, and fats) from which to choose each meal. In their place, the new model recommends that people eat the largest portion of their nourishment from whole foods (vegetables, fruits, and grains), followed by small amounts of foods from other categories including, in sequence, meats, processed foods, and oils.

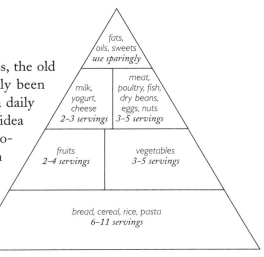

THE U.S. DAILY FOOD PYRAMID WITH RECOMMENDED SERVINGS PER DAY

*Eat Right for Your Size—Protein Consumption*

Many people eat far too little or too much protein for their body weight. But, just as Ayurvedic medicine would have recommended, modern research shows the amount of protein best for you should be based on your weight and the level of your activity.

To figure the current recommended daily allowance (RDA) of protein for your type, multiply 0.36 grams per pound of your weight. For example, a sedentary person weighing 180 pounds would have an RDA of protein nearly 65 grams per day (180 x 0.36 = 64.80 grams).

Protein is defined as an organic compound containing nitrogen, occurring in plant and animal tissue, which forms an essential part of food for animals.

## The West Discovers Prevention Foods

In addition to the above modifications recommended for the basic Western diet, the leading edge of nutritional research today focuses on discovering the many inherent antidisease properties of foods. These virtues have gone largely underresearched until recently, because Western medicine has most often turned to the pharmaceutical industry to provide cures for our ailments.

**THE HIGHEST QUALITY PROTEIN SOURCES**

Whey

Whole eggs

Egg whites

Casein—milk protein

Skim milk

Milk and cheese

Fish

Lean meat and chicken

Corn (maize)

Rice

Wheat

Oatmeal

Peanut butter

Soy flour

However, today's scientists are uncovering many complex chemical properties of foods to support the thesis that foods can be powerful preventive drugs that naturally ward off disease before it strikes. Even small changes in your diet can help prevent or alleviate illnesses like cancer, heart disease, high blood pressure, headaches, ulcers, insomnia, and low energy.

The following sections highlight significant recent findings:

*"A man may esteem himself happy when that which is his food is also his medicine."*
*—Henry David Thoreau*

### Polyphenols Against Cancer

One of the latest discoveries is polyphenols, marvelously protective chemicals found in many fruits and vegetables. According to Dr. Hans Stich of the University of British Columbia, some fruits and vegetables actually contain more polyphenols than they do the better known beta-carotene. A number of polyphenols are now confirmed to have anticancer properties, and they may also protect the cardiovascular and other body systems.

You can get polyphenols in apples, potatoes, brewed coffee, grapes, strawberries, wheat bran, plums, cherries, pears, wine (especially red wine), and in tea. Green tea packs twice the helpful phenols as black tea. Brew it for at least three minutes to get the maximum benefits.

### The Red Wine Paradox

Contrary to the common medical assumption, it turns out that drinking red wine can be beneficial to your health. Research into the tannins that give red wine their color and character reveals they contain phenolics which are an anticancer agent and act to prevent heart disease. (For you beer lovers, don't worry; it seems that beer also has a relatively large amount of phenolics from the hops.) One glass of red wine a day is sufficient.

According to the *British Medical Journal,* a study of men aged forty-five to sixty-four revealed that regular consumption of small amounts of alcohol (less than two drinks per day or fourteen per week) was correlated with a 19 percent reduction in overall mortality, including death from heart disease. In another study of women aged thirty to seventy, it was demonstrated that the risk of dying prematurely from heart disease or stroke decreased by 50 percent with wine consumption.

On the cancer front, research at the University of Illinois at Chicago indicates that red and white grapes contain a powerful anticancer agent called reservatrol (which is also present in seventy-two different plant species). Reservatrol seems to be a potent chemo-preventive agent in preventing the initiation, promotion, and progression of cancer. The University of Illinois studies show that reservatrol may interfere with the development of cancer in three ways: by blocking the action of cancer-causing agents, by causing precancerous cells to return to normal, and by inhibiting the development and growth of tumors.

As for heart disease, red wine may help to protect against it because the phenols seem to prevent deterioration of high-density lipoproteins, fatty acids that are needed for a healthy heart. The phenols in red wine are thought to act as scavengers of free radicals and toxins that would otherwise damage cell materials. Reservatrol is available in table grapes; phenols and flavanols are in grape seeds.

Furthermore, a new study reports that wine, especially red wine, helps prevent macular degeneration, a condition that causes loss of vision by affecting the retina of the eye, especially in older adults. The beneficial effect is apparently from the antioxidant components of the wine, compounds that protect the cells in the retina. One researcher involved in the study stated that even twelve glasses of wine in the course of one year will have a significant effect in preventing the disease.

The abuse of alcohol can have serious health consequences. According to John Pinto, Ph.D. of the Memorial Sloan Kettering Cancer Center in New York, alcohol abuse may be damaging to the mucus lining of the intestinal tract. Pregnant women should consult a physician regarding abstinence from alcohol during pregnancy.

*The Vegetarian Advantage—Nutraceuticals and Phytonutrients*
Studies have shown that groups of vegetarians, such as Seventh Day Adventists, have lower rates of cancer, heart disease, and

chronic diseases than the population at large. It is now believed the wide variety of fruits and vegetables they consume provides them with many natural protective agents against disease. It is not just the absence of meat, but the presence of the protective nutrients in vegetables that keeps them so healthy, according to researchers at Johns Hopkins School of Medicine, who concluded that a phytochemical found in broccoli appears to help protect against breast cancer in animal studies.

The protective powers of food are becoming so widely recognized that one scientist, Stephen L. DeFelice, M.D., founder of the Foundation for Innovation in Medicine in New York, coined a word to describe such natural chemicals: *nutraceuticals*. Nutraceuticals refers to any natural substances found in plant or animal foods that act as protective or healing agents.

One of the largest classes of nutraceuticals is called *phytonutrients*, referring to those chemicals found exclusively in plants. The chart on the following page lists the most important phytonutrients that have thus far been identified and their preventive actions.

The simplest—and best—way to harvest the benefits of the phytonutrients is to eat a wide variety of fruits and vegetables. While lower saturated fat and increased fiber play a role in the vegetarian's healthful lifestyle, it is now evident these pharmacologically protective agents—the phytonutrients in their diet of vegetables, fruits, legumes, nuts, and other plant foods—provide a potent force in counteracting cellular assaults that foster disease.

### Anticancer Vegetables

Cruciferous vegetables—which include broccoli, cabbage, and kale—are those that have flowers with four petals in the shape of a cross. In addition to their flowery cross they all share natural chemicals that counteract the destructiveness of the carcinogens in our environment.

Anticancer foods are not just folk medicine, but have been proven by meticulous scientific experiments. In one study on colon cancer, men who ate the most vegetables had the lowest rate of the disease. And among the vegetables they ate the most, cabbage was

## TWELVE ANTICANCER VEGETABLES

Broccoli

Kale

Brussels sprouts

Kohlrabi

Cabbage

Mustard

Cauliflower

Radish

Cress

Rutabaga

Horseradish

Turnip

PHYTONUTRIENTS

| Phytonutrient | Sources | Effects |
|---|---|---|
| Phytosterols | Plant oils, corn, sesame, soy, safflower, pumpkin, wheat | Inhibit uptake of cholesterol from foods, and block hormonal role in cancers. |
| Phytoestrogens | Soy products, alfalfa sprouts | Aid menopausal symptoms and may block some cancers. |
| Lycopene | Tomatoes and tomato sauce | Protect against prostate cancer and helps block UVA and UVB rays. |
| Capsaicin | Red chili peppers | Help prevent carcinogens from binding with DNA in the body's cells. |
| Catechins | Green and black tea | Active in reducing the risk of cancer in the gastrointestinal tract. |
| Sulfur compounds | Onions and all kinds of garlic | Lower blood pressure, improve immune system response, fight infections and parasites, lower cholesterol and reduce triglycerides (bad cholesterol). |
| Ascorbic acid | Citrus fruits, broccoli, and most fruits and vegetables | Bind iron, thus preventing it from becoming a cancer-causing pre-oxidant. |
| Fiber lignans | Soybeans, flaxseed, nuts | Inhibit the growth of tumors. |
| Fiber pectins | Prunes, plums, pears, apples | Improve colon health; encourage beneficial intestinal flora. |
| Protease inhibitors | Soybeans and soy products, eggs, cereals, and potatoes | Protect the body against the negative effects of radiation and free radical damage, and prevent the activation of certain genes that cause cancer. |

king. Laboratory studies show that cabbage contains active dithi-olthiones, which defeat the nefarious effects of cancer promoters in the body. Meanwhile, other studies are adding additional information that cruciferous vegetables also protect against cancers of the lung, esophagus, larynx, prostate, and bladder.

### ANTICANCER CAROTENOIDS

*Apricots*

*Dark green lettuce*

*Broccoli*

*Spinach*

*Brussels sprouts*

*Squash*

*Cabbage*

*Sweet potatoes*

*Carrots*

*Tomatoes*

*Kale*

### Carotene Vegetables

Another category of vegetables that seem to act as anticancer agents are those rich in carotenes, chemicals that give them orange or red tints. (Some of these vegetables are more green than orange because chlorophyl covers the warmer colors below the surface.) As mentioned earlier, there are some five hundred carotenoids, the best known being beta-carotene. Vegetables act as antioxidants, agents that protect against the formation of free radicals, which are loose molecules that attack cell membranes and damage our RNA and DNA, causing our cells to deteriorate. Free radicals are implicated in the aging process, as well as potential factors associated with heart disease, cancers, skin problems, and autoimmune diseases.

### Olive Oil

While the Western diet is far too rich in fat, olive oil has emerged from recent research as the safest of all the edible fats. The difference between olive oil and other fats is that oleic acid, the predominant fatty acid in olive oil, is metabolized very easily in the body. In fact, it has been shown that olive oil reduces the low-density lipoproteins (LDL), the bad cholesterol while raising the high-density lipoproteins (HDL), the good cholesterol. Olive oil also lowers blood pressure, thins the blood, and lowers the risk of death from all causes. Olive oil does not have the cardiovascular risk of saturated fats, or the cancer risks of polyunsaturated oils.

The best kind of olive oil to use is labeled extra virgin, which is oil produced by merely crushing and squeezing the highest quality olives. Extra virgin olive oil is the best source of the heart-protecting and disease-fighting chemicals found in the oil. Olive oil can be used in cooking, salad dressings, and other foods that require oil.

Olive oil has been a staple of the diet among Mediterranean peoples for four thousand years. For this reason, one of the most respected dietary guidelines recommended today is called the Mediterranean diet. This diet is composed mostly of fruits and vegetables, whole grain breads and pastas, fish, and olive oil, with only moderate amounts of red meat.

### Good Fat / Bad Fat

It's understandable if you're confused about the difference among fats, including oils. Here's a rundown on the three main categories:

- *Saturated fats*—Natural sources of saturated fats are red meats, unskinned poultry, whole milk products, and the tropical oils made from palm and coconut. Heart experts have warned us to avoid or cut down on these sources. Man-made sources of saturated fat include margarine, solid vegetable shortening, and all foods made with partially hydrogenated vegetable oils. Hydrogenated oils are artifi-cially processed until they become saturated with hydrogen. This makes them solid or semisolid at room temperature, and increases their shelf life, but also produces trans-fatty acids, or TFAs, an unnatural and toxic form of fat. TFAs in the diet damage the regulatory mechanisms of the body, significantly compromising the healing system. Nutritional experts recommend you eliminate from your diet all mar-garine and solid shortening and products made from them.

- *Polyunsaturated fats*—Polyunsaturated fats remain truly liq-uid at room temperature. They include corn, soy, sesame, sunflower, and safflower oils. At one time, safflower oil, the most unsaturated of all the vegetable oils, was considered a healthy choice. Recent studies have changed this opinion because polyunsaturated oils are chemically unstable. They can react with oxygen, resulting in the creation of toxic compounds. Most commercial brands of polyunsaturated vegetable oils have been extracted with heat and solvents that promote the formation of TFAs.

*"Only one tablespoon of olive oil can wipe out the cholesterol-raising effects of two eggs. Four or five tablespoons of olive oil daily dramatically improves the blood profiles of heart attack patients. And two-thirds of a tablespoon daily lowered blood pressure in men."*

—*Jean Carper,*
The Food Pharmacy

- *Monounsaturated fats*—There are four monounsaturated vegetable oils: Olive oil has the most evidence of health benefits, the longest record of successful use by large populations, and is the most highly recommended.

  Canola oil is made from rapeseed, a relative of the mustard family. The name is a contraction of Canadian oil, as it was developed in Canada. Only organic and expeller-pressed canola oil found in health food stores is recommended by health experts, as commercial brands may have pesticide residues or problems stemming from the methods used for extraction.

  Peanut oil has more polyunsaturated oils than olive oil.

  Avocado oil is more expensive than olive oil.

### Fish and Omega-3 Fatty Acids

Omega-3 fatty acids are found in oily fishes from cold northern waters, as well as in flax and hemp plants, and in a wild green plant called purslane. These fatty acids are highly unsaturated, and appear to have many health benefits. Studies show that they may protect against cancer, degenerative changes in cells and tissues, abnormal blood clotting, and inflammation. The recommended diet includes three servings a week of northern fish: sardines, herring, mackerel, bluefish, salmon, and albacore tuna. (Salmon, sardines, and herring seem to be the best sources.)

If you don't like fish, you can get the omega-3 fatty acids from flax oil, seeds, or meal. A tablespoon of the oil or two tablespoons of the flax meal each day, when used with food, are a good source. Flax seeds are rich in omega-3s, and can be ground in a coffee grinder. You can also use hemp oil, which is available in many health food stores. A tablespoon per day can be mixed with olive oil or salad dressing. Purslane, a Mediterranean plant, is not so easily obtained in stores, but can be grown in your garden.

### The Serendipity of Soybeans

In the food pharmacopoeia, special mention needs to be made of soybeans. As a protein source, they are as good as meat proteins.

In addition they have a list of health benefits that include:

- Protecting against cancer risks

- Protecting against cardiovascular system disease

- Lowering cholesterol

- Reducing triglycerides

- Regulating blood sugar

- Improving colon function and health

Soybeans are an excellent source of the anticancer protease inhibitors. By promoting a healthy colon, they are also protective against other problems such as diverticulitis, hemorrhoids, and constipation. A soybean paste soup, called *miso* in Japan, has been shown to reduce the risk of stomach cancer by one-third in Japanese men and women who ate one bowl of miso soup a day.

Dr. David Jenkins of the University of Toronto calls soybeans a good way to control blood sugar, and to promote the desirable flat blood sugar response. Eating soybeans in place of dairy and meat products reduced LDL (bad) cholesterol from 15 to 20 percent in Italian adults and children. Soy fiber mixed into baked goods can bring down cholesterol, as can textured soybean protein. Some researchers believe a soybean diet can even counteract the bad effects of fat in your diet. Dr. David Klurfeld's research suggests that if you eat half your protein in soybean based foods, you can revitalize your arteries, making them less susceptible to stroke or heart disease.

You can find soybeans in many forms today to replace some of the protein you might otherwise get from meat or dairy products. There is soy milk, which can be used as a milk substitute. The best soy milk is found in the refrigerated dairy case at a health food store. Soy powder mixes easily into blender drinks. There is soy flour, and roasted soybeans called soy nuts. Tofu, a soft, white product made from curdled soy milk, is an excellent source of protein, and can be put in a blender with fruit to start the day. There are also fermented soybeans (tempeh), soybean flakes, soybean sprouts, and textured vegetable protein. Soybean products simulate meat in vegetable burgers, sausage, bacon bits, and other packaged foods. Medical experts consider soy protein as good as meat protein.

## Powerful Benefits from Foods

According to Stephanie Beling, M.D., there are several highly beneficial food groups she calls power foods. Here are some of them:

POWER FOODS

| Food Group | Beneficial Effects |
|---|---|
| Garlic & onions | Infection and cancer fighters, good for the heart, anti-inflammatory, reduces LDL (bad) cholesterol. |
| Soy & soy products | Anticancer, especially to prevent hormone related cancers of the breast, ovaries, and prostate. Reduces the risk of heart disease. |
| Whole grains | A good energy source. Helps to aid in elimination and prevent colon cancer. Lowers cholesterol. Improves insulin sensitivity. |
| Leafy green & cruciferous vegetables | Stimulates cancer fighting enzymes. Neutralizes harmful free radicals. Controls hormones. |
| Red, yellow, & orange fruits & vegetables | Prevents degenerative diseases, including diabetes, heart disease and arthritis. Protects vision. A good source of antioxidants. |
| Nuts & seeds | Anti-inflammatory, helpful in elimination; lowers cholesterol, stimulates enzymes that detoxify carcinogens, and enhances the immune system. |
| Beans & legumes in general | Helps with a healthy digestion and good elimination. Lowers LDL cholesterol. Alters harmful hormone pathways, and has cancer fighting enzymes. |
| Mushrooms | Anti-tumor, anti-viral; enhances the immune system. |
| Sea vegetables | Increases metabolism, minimizes heavy metal toxicity, and helps build strong bones. |

## Natural Antibiotics

We usually think of antibiotics as drugs that combat infections, but it turns out that nature has created her own powerful antibiotics for us. One of the best is cranberry juice, which has been shown to be an effective antibiotic in the urinary tract. Cranberry juice is often recommended for men with prostate infections, and for women with urinary tract infections.

Garlic and onions are natural antibiotics, in addition to being hypocholesterolemic (cholesterol reducing), and anticoagulating (blood clot preventing). Now proven in laboratories, the health benefits of garlic have been at work for years in the popular Mediterranean diet.

## Chapter Recap

- Western medicine has recently adopted many concepts of preventive nutrition, in line with the alternative traditions. New scientific discoveries have brought about a greater understanding of the role food plays in maintaining health and fighting disease.

- Eat whole grains, whole fruits, and vegetables rather than trying to get all of your higher nutrition from supplemental capsules. Try to eat a healthy diet with appropriate amounts of food from each part of the pyramid each day. Make sure most of your intake consists of grains, fruits, and vegetables, with lesser amounts of meats, sugars, and fats.

- The Nutraceutical Revolution has shown that many food substances act as healing agents, especially in preventing cancer and heart disease. Some foods contain agents that act as drugs.

- Focus on foods with phytonutrients, as well as anticancer vegetables and anticancer carotenoids.

- Use olive oil more than polyunsaturated oils. Avoid saturated fats including margarine.

- Eat three servings of cold water oily fish (like salmon or tuna) per week to obtain healthy omega-3 fatty acids.

- Consider modifying your diet to include soybean products for your protein source rather than meat or dairy products.

*Recommended Reading*

Morgan, Dr. Brian L. G. *Nutrition Prescription.* New York: Crown Publishers, 1987.

Carper, Jean. *The Food Pharmacy.* New York: Bantam, 1989.

# Nutritional Supplements

*T*his chapter examines the best known sources of vitality from the natural healing traditions, as well as the latest discoveries in the area of vitamin and mineral therapy.

## Ayurvedic Concepts of Vitality

The Ayurvedic tradition teaches that food is a key element in maintaining vitality and optimum health. The most important recommendations from Ayurveda are those that focus on eating according to your constitution, as discussed in Chapter 1. The goal of the Ayurvedic diet is to eat those foods that balance your dosha and to avoid those foods that aggravate it.

Ayurveda also teaches specific principles to ensure the preservation of vitality. In *Ayurvedic Secrets to Longevity & Total Health*, Peter Anselmo and James S. Brooks, M.D. outline some of the most important concepts of this ancient tradition:

- Full and complete digestion is critical to enhancing vitality. For this reason food should be fresh and natural, as free from chemicals, pesticides, and fertilizers as possible. Use the best quality food that you can afford.

- It is best to follow a vegetarian diet. Favor cooked food over raw, because it is easier to digest and will contribute more to your energy. Raw fruit is an exception to the cooking rule.

- Milk should be taken separately from the regular meal. Milk combines well with cereals and whole grains. It is best to heat milk first, and to add a small amount of turmeric, ginger powder, or cardamom to improve its digestibility.

- Start each meal with a small amount of fresh or pickled ginger, to stimulate digestive juices.

- Avoid ice cold foods and drinks because they impede and impair digestion. Ayurveda teaches that their coldness tends to put out the digestive fire.

- Fried foods should be eaten only occasionally, and only by someone whose digestive fire is strong, as the digestive enzymes have difficulty breaking them down into their nutrients.

- At night, avoid heavy foods, such as buttermilk, cheese, yogurt, and ice cream. They are hard to digest and tend to produce ama which are impurities.

  People should avoid overeating. In the Ayurvedic view, maintaining the right weight for your constitution greatly influences your vitality.

## Tonics and Traditional Chinese Medicine

Ancient Chinese medicine was perhaps the first system to promote the use of *tonics*—foods or substances that help make an individual stronger, healthier, and more disease-resistant. Tonics were not medicines for ill people, but supplements that all people could take to increase their vitality, strength, endurance, and all-around good health. In short, one might say tonics were the earliest version of nutritional supplements.

The leading tonic in ancient China was ginseng, an herbal root growing naturally in many temperate forested areas of China. It is estimated that ginseng has been in use in China for five thousand years, and was discovered through medical observation to act as a tonic, just as many other herbs were discovered to have culinary or medicinal value. In ancient Chinese medical literature, it was thought that ginseng acquired the nutrients from the ground in which it was grown, and these nutrients are what caused it to boost one's energy, relieve fatigue, and build resistance to disease. The herb was used especially among older people who benefited from its healthful properties to live longer and more productive lives. Ginseng was so prized in ancient China that the best roots were reserved for the aristocracy and the emperor. Even among the general population, the cost of a small root of average quality was expensive.

### GINSENG—THE KING OF HERBS

*The word ginseng originates from the Chinese words jen and shen. Shen means root, and the root is the most useful and potent part of this plant, not the stem or leaves. Jen means man and ginseng has the unusual, if not humorous, property of having its root resemble a man's body. A mature ginseng root consists of a main stalk that looks like a male's torso, and there are usually several small shoots that look like arms, legs—and sometimes even what could look like male genitalia. Some plants even have facial markings on the top portion of the root. This resemblance of ginseng to a man is one reason the herb has often been associated with aphrodisiacs in many cultures. In ancient China it was believed that a plant's appearance was an indication of what part of the body it would benefit. (In other words, if the ginseng looked like a male with a penis, men believed that it could be used to stimulate sexual desire.) As it turns out, modern science now knows that ginseng has specific healthful effects on the hormonal system that can help to moderate the body's stress reaction, improve mental performance, and even enhance sexual performance.*

The most common method of preparing ginseng was to gather the roots in the fall. Even thousands of years ago, it was respected that roots had to mature and be at least seven years old to have medicinal value. The roots were then either dried in the air (in which case the skin was peeled off) or steamed (in which case the skin was on). The drying process protected the roots from rot and insects and allowed them to be stored for long periods of time. The dried peeled root was called white ginseng because of its color, whereas a steamed root was called red ginseng because the steaming process turns the skin red. Whichever drying method was used, a ginseng root was then sliced and boiled in water several times to make a brew that could be drunk like a tea. Sometimes the root was pulverized into powder that could be added to water to make tea. Another common method of preparing ginseng was to soak a mashed-up root in a mixture of water and alcohol such as vodka to make an alcohol extract or tincture, which lasted longer than the cold water brew, and was easier to make. The tincture was then drunk in small amounts, straight. Another common way to prepare ginseng was to throw slices of the root into soup.

### Ginseng and the Modern Adaptogen Theory

Ginseng usage originated in China though other varieties of the same plant were found in many locales. As it did in China, ginseng became a staple of the diet in ancient India, Japan, Korea, and Vietnam, often taken as a tincture or in tea. In the 1700s, ginseng became popular among Europeans and colonial Americans. It is known that many tribes of Native Americans used the American species of the ginseng plant for the same purposes as the Chinese. Today, ginseng is still considered the king of Chinese herbs, and is used by millions of people throughout the world.

Although the medical value of ginseng was often denigrated as folklore, recent scientific research validates its healthful properties—and the concept that ginseng is a tonic. The leading edge of ginseng research was started in the 1950s when two Soviet scientists, Professor N.V. Lazarev and Itskovity I. Brekhman of the Institute of Physiology and Pharmacology in Vladisvostok, began looking for naturally available plants and foods they believed could help people maintain good health at all times. Lazarev dubbed these substances *adaptogens*, because he thought they would help the body adapt or adjust to any stressful condition. Lazarev specifically defined three criteria that adaptogens had to fulfill:

- They had to be innocuous, i.e., cause minimal disruption in the functions of an organism.

- They had to be non-specific in action, meaning that they must increase resistance to a wide variety of physical, chemical, and biochemical factors.

- They had to cause a normalizing action that brings the body back to balance.

Recent sophisticated scientific analysis has discovered that ginseng actually does contain several active ingredients with measurable pharmacological and metabolic effects on many parts of the body, particularly the central nervous system and the hormonal system. These ingredients are called *saponins*, which are large sugarlike compounds, just like those found in many types of plants. While the various species of ginseng contain different amounts of these saponins, they all have the same general effect of helping the body moderate its natural response to stress. A number of experiments suggest that ginseng strengthens the adrenal glands and possibly also affects the brain center, called the hypothalamus, and the pituitary gland. These combine to regulate the flow of adrenaline in the body. The less adrenaline flowing through the body, the less stress the body experiences.

In the twentieth century, the concept of tonics or adaptogens to revitalize the body and mind is only recently accepted by conventional Western medicine. Most Western scientists are still attempting to understand and define the term more precisely. Any definition acceptable to the West must be put in scientific terms. As a result, some scientists studying adaptogens recently attempted to define them as substances that perform the following functions:

- Support the hormonal system

- Enable cells to get more energy and to utilize it more efficiently

- Strengthen the brain centers that regulate our biorhythms

- Help cells eliminate toxins and by-products of cellular activity

Western researchers are now recognizing that herbs, food sources, and other natural products are adaptogens, including red wine and other foods containing phenolics. They appear to rid the body of toxins and protect HDL levels in the blood.

In addition, science now regards two natural human activities as potential adaptogens:

- *Exercise*—In the last decade, research discovered that vigorous exercise causes the mind to release a cascade of healthful hormones, called endorphins, that flow through the body, reinvigorating many bodily systems. Recent research indicates that endorphins contribute to a greatly enhanced immune response in the body as well as an increase in physical and mental energy. As you have probably heard, people who jog or engage in vigorous workouts say they almost feel high from the experience.

- *Laughter*—Another surprising human function that appears to have adaptogenic properties is laughter. Following the research of Norman Cousins, who studied the role of laughter in mitigating cancer, many scientists believe laughter creates significant hormonal changes in the body that heightens the immune system's response to disease, as well as increases both mental and physical performance.

## *The Western Approach to Supplements*

Over the last thirty years, a growing awareness has developed that many people in Western industrialized countries do not receive adequate nutrition, even if they seem to eat enough food. A variety of reasons can explain the problem:

- *Freshness*—The majority of people in modern societies throughout the world often lack access to fresh produce, and lack the time to prepare it in the ways to preserve its nutritional value. According to the National Center for Health Statistics, only 9 percent of adults in the U.S. eat enough fresh produce to get the recommended daily requirements of vitamins and minerals.

- *Overfarming*—Farming methods now in use often deplete foods of their nutritional value. The overuse of soil, for example, reduces the nutrient levels of food grown in them. Even with chemical fertilizer added to the soil, the quality of the nutrients suffers. Some of the soils in which crops are grown have been especially depleted of trace minerals like iodine or selenium. Selenium is an antioxidant that protects cells against cancer, toxic chemicals, radiation, heavy metals, and other free radical damage.

- *Shipping time*—The time between harvesting the foods and eating them can often run into days or weeks, further sapping the foods of the natural nutrients. Dr. Michael Colgon of the Rockefeller Institute has performed studies that reveal that many of the oranges sold in local supermarkets today contain absolutely no vitamin C. This is because oranges are often picked long before they mature so they can be packed, stored, and shipped to arrive looking fresh. They are then ripened with the use of a gas, in many instances, and stored for fairly long periods of time. Oranges and other fruits can lose significant amounts of nutrients starting the day after they are picked. Even people committed to a healthy lifestyle who eat large amounts of commercially produced fruits and vegetables rarely get sufficient quantities of many of the essential vitamins and minerals in their diet.

- *Toxins*—Modern society seems to expose us to more and more toxins that cause cancer and other diseases. This constant exposure increases our need for fresh fruits and vegetables which contain the nutrients needed to fight free radicals, the highly reactive molecules that damage cells and their DNA.

As a result, many Western doctors who subscribe to a strong preventive view of medicine now recommend that most people add vitamin and mineral supplements to their daily regimen.

### The Vital Vitamin

Vitamins are micronutrients necessary for life. A dictionary defines vitamins as: "Organic substances present in many foods and essential to the nutrition of man and other animals." Vitamins act as *cofactors,* or regulators, of many metabolic processes essential to life. In the early 1900s, vitamins were called accessory factors, but by 1911 researchers concluded that they were much more than mere accessories, they were in fact *vital,* crucial to life. In 1920 the term *vitamin* was created to recognize their vital nature.

The complete removal of one or more vitamins from your diet, if continued for a long enough time, will result in illness. Fortunately, completely removing a vitamin from one's diet is very

### U.S. ADULT RECOMMENDED DAILY ALLOWANCES FOR VITAMINS

| *Vitamin* | *Quantities* |
| --- | --- |
| Vitamin A | 4,000–5,000 IU |
| Vitamin B1 (thiamine) | 1.2–1.5 mg |
| Vitamin B2 (riboflavin) | 1.4–1.8 mg |
| Vitamin B3 (niacin) | 16–20 mg |
| Vitamin B5 (pantothenic acid) | 4–7 mg |
| Vitamin B6 (pyroxidane) | 2.0–2.5 mg |
| Vitamin B12 (cobalamin) | 3.0–4.0 mcg |
| Folic Acid (folate, folacin) | 400 mcg |
| Biotin | 150–300 mcg |
| Vitamin C | 60 mg |
| Vitamin D | 400 IU |
| Vitamin E | 12–15 IU |
| Vitamin K | 65 mcg |

hard to do, except in a laboratory. However, it is not difficult to become deficient in one or more vitamins if your eating habits are poor or if you eat mostly processed foods that lack the full range of vitamins found in whole foods. Vitamin deficiencies are serious, as they can cause health problems.

Vitamins are found in foods, although vitamin D can also be made by the body through sunlight exposed to the skin. To rely on foods for all your vitamin needs as some experts advocate, you would have to eat large amounts of fresh vegetables and fresh fruits, and eat them mostly raw. Fish, poultry, lean meats, whole unrefined grains, whole grain cereals, and some dairy products do supply other vitamins.

The problem is, there are many factors that influence how vitamin rich or vitamin poor our foods are, including:

- Where the foods were grown or produced

- What standards were used to produce the foods

- The nutrients (or lack of them) in the soil

- The presence of added chemicals and pesticides

- When they were harvested and how long they were stored

- If and for how long they were cooked

Furthermore, outside influences—such as air and water pollution and the level of toxic materials in the environment—as well as individual influences—such as your level of stress or physical and mental problems—can significantly alter your need for additional vitamins. For all of these reasons, many alternative Western doctors now recommend you supplement your diet with vitamins as insurance against the known problems and your unknown health needs.

### *What Vitamins Do*
- *Vitamin A*—Necessary for night vision and for the health of the mucous membranes, which include the mouth, nose,

and digestive system. It works to build bones, blood, and teeth. It maintains the health of the sex organs and works to energize the immune system. Sources of vitamin A are vegetables, found as beta-carotene and other carotenoids. These nutrients are converted in the body to vitamin A in the amounts that are needed. Another source of vitamin A is fish liver oil. Some people, such as diabetics, cannot assimilate beta-carotene, and use fish liver oil instead.

THE B VITAMINS

*Thiamine (vitamin B1)*

*Riboflavin (B2)*

*Niacin, also called niaci-
namide (B3)*

*Pyridoxine (B6)*

*Cobalamin (B12)*

*Biotin*

*Choline*

*Inositol*

*Folic acid, also called folate*

*Para-aminobenzoic acid
(PABA)*

*Pantothenic acid (calcium
pantothenate—B5)*

- *The B vitamins*—a family of supplements available individually but best taken together.

According to John D. Kirschmann, author of the *Nutrition Almanac*, the vitamin B family provides the body with energy by converting carbohydrates into glucose, which the body then burns. They are also vital in the metabolism of fats and protein. In addition, the B vitamins are necessary for the normal functioning of the nervous system and may be the single most important factor for the health of the nerves. They are also essential for the maintenance of muscle tone in the gastrointestinal tract and for the health of the skin, hair, eyes, mouth, and liver.

However, note that the B vitamins are all water soluble, which means any amounts not needed by the body are not stored, but are secreted in your urine. As a result, the B vitamins need to be resupplied daily via food sources and/or vitamin supplements. Without this replenishment, a deficiency of one or more B vitamins can cause nerve disorders, stress, fatigue, anemia, insomnia, digestive problems, and allergies.

- *Vitamin C*—Most animals are able to make their own vitamin C, but humans cannot. Some researchers have speculated that, thousands of years ago, humans lived in an environment where vitamin C was abundant in the plant food, and they consumed from 2,000 mg to 3,000 mg daily in their diet, perhaps making it unnecessary to manufacture their own. Whether that interesting idea is true or not, we may never know as it is shrouded in the mist of time. What is clear though is that today's humans must take in vitamin C on a daily basis, as it is water soluble.

Vitamin C is also known as ascorbic acid, from its ability to prevent the disease of scurvy. Most of us have heard the story of how scurvy was the scourge of the British naval fleet until James Lind discovered that drinking citrus fruit juices would completely prevent it. What is not widely known is that Lind's advice was not heeded until forty years had gone by from the time he first discovered and demonstrated its effectiveness!

> ### TRY TIMED RELEASE FOR WATER SOLUBLE VITAMINS
>
> *The family of B vitamins, which are water soluble and can't be stored in the body, can be purchased in timed release tablets. The advantage of timed release vitamins is when they are released gradually, they can be absorbed more effectively by the cells of the body. More of the active ingredients are absorbed, and the kidneys eliminate less. Another strategy is to take them at intervals during the day, in other words, to divide the doses. This is also more effective than one large dose of water soluble vitamins.*

Vitamin C has been shown to have a powerful role in the prevention of many health problems including infections, the common cold, and even cancer. It also protects against the effects of pollution and is a major member of the antioxidant team that controls the damage caused by free radicals. It helps maintain collagen, the connective tissue that holds the body together, and has a role in longevity and a healthier old age. A deficiency of vitamin C can result in susceptibility to infections, bruising, bleeding gums, and atherosclerosis.

Sources of vitamin C are fresh fruits and vegetables. Ascorbic acid can be taken in powder form. Some medical experts recommend calcium ascorbate powder, which is non-acidic and supplies calcium. One quarter teaspoon of powder supplies 1,000 mg of vitamin C. The recommended daily allowance (RDA) for vitamin C is from 50–100 mg per day. However, many nutritionists recommend even greater amounts, called the supplement dosage recommended (SDR), from 250–2,000 mg per day. Vitamin C is best taken at intervals throughout the day, or in time-release form to avoid irritating the stomach. It works well when taken with other vitamins and minerals. Acid sensitive individuals should consult a health practitioner about higher doses.

### VITAMIN C AND BIOFLAVONOIDS

*Bioflavonoids are substances found in the leaves, stems, flowers, fruits, and roots of most plants. They are neither vitamins nor minerals, but they have specific health benefits, especially in combination with vitamin C. While there are more than eight hundred flavonoids distributed in plants, the primary bioflavonoids often combined in vitamin supplements are citrus bioflavonoids. These are found abundantly in the white rind of oranges and other citrus fruits. The three bioflavonoids most often used are rutin, quercetin, and hesperidin. They protect vitamin C from oxidation, which destroys it, and have other healthful benefits such as strengthening blood vessels and constricting the capillaries. A deficiency of bioflavonoids can result in colds, bruising, and nosebleeds.*

*Sources of bioflavonoids include citrus fruits, black currants, cherries, buckwheat, green pepper, grapes, garlic, and tomatoes. (When preparing fresh citrus fruits, cut away the outer skin, while leaving on the white rind that is underneath, to increase your intake of these healthful nutrients.)*

*You can also buy vitamin C tablets with bioflavonoids included. This is helpful, because flavonoids play an important role in the body's conversion of vitamin C into its metabolically active form, so the cells can use it. It has been observed clinically that flavonoids improve the therapeutic action of vitamin C.*

- *Vitamin D*—The vitamin we can make in our own body through the action of the sunshine on our skin. However, there is an impediment to this ability, as you need to expose a lot of skin to sunlight for long periods of the day, on a regular basis. When an oil forms on your skin, you then have to wait for it to be absorbed, rather than wash it off by swimming or showering. Unfortunately, research has shown that exposure to sun is dangerous for the skin. For this reason, it is best to obtain the majority of your vitamin D through food and supplements.

Vitamin D is important in the absorption of calcium and phosphorus, which are needed to grow strong bones and teeth. The synthesized form of vitamin D (called D2), which is added to milk, aids the absorption of minerals. Vitamin D also affects the nerves, thyroid, and blood clotting functions. A deficiency of vitamin D can result in soft bones and teeth, poor metabolism, nervousness, and muscular weakness.

Sources of vitamin D are salmon, tuna, herring, cod liver oil, other fish liver oils, egg yolks, liver, and sunshine on your skin.

• *Vitamin E*—The principal protector of the body's cells against the ravages of free radicals. In its basic function as an antioxidant it prevents the oxidation of HDLs, the good unsaturated fatty acids, by trapping the free radicals which otherwise would destroy them. Oxidation of the unsaturated fatty acids can lead to cell damage. Vitamin E, by protecting the body cells in this way, has an important role in keeping the body healthier and slowing down the aging process. It is an important nutrient for the heart by increasing blood flow to the heart and thinning the blood through retarding of blood clotting. It also functions in the maintenance of cells, blood, capillaries, muscles, nerves, lungs, hair, and skin. A deficiency of vitamin E can affect the systems it protects and maintains.

Sources of vitamin E are cold pressed vegetable oil, seeds, nuts, eggs, soybeans, dark green vegetables, whole grains, wheat germ oil, and organ meats.

• *Vitamin K*—Necessary to growth, cell longevity, blood coagulation, liver function, and bile absorption. A deficiency can cause prolonged bleeding.

Sources of vitamin K are green vegetables, kelp, alfalfa, eggs, milk, soybeans, and yogurt.

### Minerals—Partners in Health

Minerals are also essential to your health, as vital as vitamins are to your overall physical and mental well-being. In fact, vitamins do you no good without minerals. It is only in the presence of minerals that vitamins are absorbed and utilized. Vitamins and minerals are co-partners; they are both essential to your body's growth, maintenance, and function. (Not all vitamins have mineral

U.S. ADULT RECOMMENDED DAILY ALLOWANCES

| Mineral | Quantities |
|---------|-----------|
| Calcium | 800–1,200 mg |
| Chromium | 50–200 mcg |
| Copper | 2–3 mg |
| Iodine | 150 mcg |
| Iron | 10–18 mg |
| Magnesium | 300–350 mg |
| Manganese | 2.5–5.0 mg |
| Phosphorus | 900–1,200 mg |
| Selenium | 55–200 mcg |
| Zinc | 15 mg |

cofactors.) Together, they are catalysts that assist in the formation and function of enzymes. Minerals work better when all the necessary ones are present in the body.

When it comes to getting minerals, you are totally dependent on obtaining them through your diet and any supplements you may take. The body does not make minerals.

Here is a list of the minerals you need:

- *Calcium*—builds the bones and teeth of the body, in concert with phosphorus, magnesium, and vitamins A and C. It works with the heart in muscle growth and muscle movement. It also helps you sleep when you take it at night. Calcium is often combined in supplements with vitamin D to increase absorption. Combined with vitamin C, calcium becomes calcium ascorbate. Take it in divided doses throughout the day.

- *Chloride*—assists in maintaining the correct balance of fluids and electrolytes in the body. It has a role in the maintenance of tendons and joints, and in the detoxifying function of the liver. Combined with potassium or sodium, it is necessary for the production of hydrochloric acid in the stomach, which is required for mineral assimilation and protein digestion.

• *Chromium*—an essential trace mineral that promotes the efficient function of the hormone your body produces called insulin, where it is a co-factor with insulin to remove glucose from the blood into the cells. It is essential for the utilization of sugar. Chromium works with numerous other enzymes and hormones, and stimulates the function of enzymes involved in the synthesis of fatty acids, cholesterol, and protein, and in the metabolism of energy.

• *Copper*—involved in keeping the natural color of the hair. It is part of many enzymes, and aids in protein metabolism, healing, and the development of bone, connective tissue, nervous and brain tissue. It works in concert with vitamin C to form elastin.

• *Iodine*—an essential nutrient for the thyroid gland, which regulates the rate of metabolism, energy production, and body weight.

• *Iron*—important in the creation of healthy red blood cells. The better your blood, the better your resistance to stress and disease. Iron needs vitamin C to be absorbed from the intestinal tract. For this reason, iron-rich foods are best eaten with citrus juices. Iron also is the transporter of oxygen, in hemoglobin, to all parts of the body.

In the diets of American women, iron and calcium are the two minerals found most to be deficient. Calcium is needed to prevent osteoporosis in men and women.

• *Magnesium*—a mineral that works with well with calcium. The two are often found combined in supplements, with a ratio of about twice the calcium for the amount of magnesium. Magnesium performs many functions; it is a natural tranquilizer. It helps to regulate heart rhythms, cholesterol metabolism, and blood sugar levels. In concert with calcium, it builds up the bones and teeth.

- *Manganese*—A nerve and brain nutrient. It is found in enzymes that metabolize (break down) fats, proteins, and carbohydrates. It helps in the digestion and utilization of fats, when combined with choline, a B vitamin.

- *Phosphorus*—Needed for healthy nerves and efficient mental activity. It is important to maintaining a balance between acid and alkaline in the blood and body tissues. It works with calcium to grow strong teeth and bones and plays an important role in the production of energy. It functions in the utilization of carbohydrates, fats, and proteins for growth, maintenance, and repair at the cellular level.

- *Potassium*—Important in controlling the functions of the nervous system, kidneys, and heart muscles. It works to maintain the acid-alkaline balance in the tissues and blood. It promotes the secretion of hormones. One of potassium's main functions is to help regulate water balance in the body. Potassium, found mostly within cell walls, does this by working in concert with sodium, found mostly outside cell walls. Together they form a sodium/potassium pump to move fluids and nutrients into and out of cells.

- *Selenium*—Considered a trace mineral, selenium is an important antioxidant, controlling the activity of free radicals. It may help to delay aging and prevent hardening of tissues. Along with vitamin E, it protects cell membranes and it is recommended that you take the two together.

- *Sulfur*—Essential in forming body tissues. It is necessary for healthy skin, hair, and nails. Sulfur assists in tissue respiration, bile secretion from the liver, and the overall balance of the body.

- *Zinc*—A familiar mineral to many who take it to
  resist viral infections. A newer type of zinc, called zinc
  picolinate is now recommended by nutritional experts.
  The RDA for zinc is 15 mg, and the SDR is from
  20–50 mg. In addition to its infection-fighting properties, zinc assists in digesting food, maintaining
  blood sugar levels, and healing wounds. Along with
  pumpkin seed oil and the natural herb saw palmetto,
  zinc is often recommended by doctors in the alleviation of prostate conditions.

### Supplements in Chinese Medicine

Sometimes the medical traditions reverse roles. The scientific
research of Western medicine on vitamin and mineral
supplements, is now influencing Chinese medicine. While
Chinese medicine traditionally teaches that whole foods and
natural herbs are the best sources of nutrients, many modern
practitioners of traditional Chinese medicine now recommend
new strategies that utilize nutritional support from vitamin and
mineral supplements.

In *The Complete Book of Chinese Health & Healing,* Daniel Reid
presents the following recommended dosages of supplements
according to modern Chinese medicine.

### SUPPLEMENTS IN CHINESE MEDICINE

| Vitamin | Dosage | Western Recommendations |
| --- | --- | --- |
| Vitamin C | 3,000–6,000 mg in three doses | 300–3,000 mg |
| Vitamin E | 800–1200 IU (International Units) | 200–400 IU |
| Vitamin B complex | 50–100 mg | 50 IU |
| Beta-carotene | 25,000–50,000 IU | |
| Selenium | 250 mcg | 100–200 mcg |
| Zinc | 50 mg | 15–30 mg |

*Co-Q-10*

Coenzymes are compounds that interact with enzymes, assisting them in the performance of their biochemical functions. Many members of the B vitamin family described above act as coenzymes in metabolism.

In recent research, new attention has been directed to another coenzyme, ubiquinone, familiarly known as Coenzyme Q-10 and often abbreviated as Co-Q-10. It is a natural substance, present in most foods, that helps in the metabolism at the cellular level. According to Dr. Andrew Weil, it improves the use of oxygen at the cellular level, especially in heart muscle cells. Dr. Weil recommends taking a supplement of 60 mg once a day, with more if needed up to 200 mg per day. Some users report that Co-Q-10 also increases their aerobic endurance, i.e., their ability to function at higher heart and lung rates.

Natural sources of Co-Q-10 include spinach, alfalfa, potato, sweet potato, rice bran, whole grains, and soybeans.

### CO-Q-IO AND THE HEALTH OF YOUR GUMS

*For anyone over the age of forty, and for some younger, the health of your gums becomes an important area of preventive health care. If you are seeking to prevent periodontal disease, supplemental Co-Q-10 can help. According to Emile G. Bliznakov, M.D. in his book, The Miracle Nutrient Coenzyme Q 10, periodontal disease accounts for more lost teeth in adulthood than any other dental problem. He indicates that gum disease affects nine out of ten Americans, and one out of four persons lose all their teeth to periodontal disease by the time they reach age sixty. However, researchers have found Co-Q-10 can provide some good news for people with periodontal disease. Those patients who received Co-Q-10 as therapy have all improved in some fashion, and for some, the disease was reversible.*

*A periodontist, Dr. Edward G. Wilkinson, of the Department of Periodontics, U.S. Air Force Medical Center, Travis Air Force Base, California, performed a double-blind trial with members of the U.S. Air Force using a daily regimen of an oral supplement of 75 mg a day of Co-Q-10. "What we witnessed was, for lack of a more accurate medical phrase, not just a therapeutic treatment to alleviate symptoms, but a reversal of the disease state in some cases and a regrowth of healthy tissue. Coenzyme Q 10 is essential for every person to live. Without the presence of it, the essential healthy functioning of the cells break down. There is no energy in the cell, so in a very real sense it is dying. And this is what we see in periodontal disease. We see a lot of dead cells and inflammation of the connective tissues. It appears that most people have an adequate supply of Co-Q-10, but some people don't seem to be able to assimilate it as well as others. Periodontal tissues that are deficient in Co-Q-10 are diseased, and appear to require more Co-Q-10 to heal. I believe that persons suffering from periodontal disease could benefit from Co-Q-10 as an adjunct to routine periodontal therapy."*

Soybeans are an excellent source, both in soybean products and their oil. Among nuts, peanuts have the highest amount of Co-Q-10.

## Chapter Recap

• Ayurvedic medicine generally looks to a healthful diet as the best insurance against losing vitality and balance. It does recommend some additional foods though, such as ginger at the beginning of meals, to stimulate digestion.

• Chinese medicine believes firmly in the concept of tonics, substances that promote health and wellness regardless of one's physical state. The leading tonic is the herb ginseng. Western science is now confirming that ginseng has a measurable effect on the body's hormonal system, which appears to moderate its reaction to stress and enhance immunity.

• Farming and marketing methods can deplete foods of their nutritional value. As a result, many Western doctors now encourage preventive nutrition, recommending that people supplement their diet with vitamins and minerals to support essential cellular functions, promote immunity, and fight the disease-causing toxins that are increasing in our environment.

• Vitamins also require minerals to function effectively. Many vitamins have mineral counterparts needed to ensure that the vitamins are absorbed and utilized properly in the body.

• Coenzyme Q-10, previously known as a supplement that is good for your heart, is now known to be beneficial in maintaining the health of the gums and preventing periodontal disease, a serious concern for people over forty.

*Recommended Reading*

Bosco, Dominick. *The People's Guide to Vitamins and Minerals.* Chicago: Contemporary Books, 1989.

Lee, William H., R.P.H., Ph.D. *Vitamin Primer.* New York: Lee Press, 1995.

# *W a t e r — t h e   E l i x i r*

# *o f   L i f e*

*W*ater is the major component of the body, constituting 75 percent by proportion. The brain is approximately 85 percent water. Water makes up the majority of the body's blood, muscles, and organs. It transports oxygen to the body's trillions of cells. It conducts the subtle electrical currents that fly through the body, which we can measure in the heart by an EKG test, and in the brain by the EEG test. Chronic dehydration, therefore, is a major stressor to the body. Dehydration weakens the kidneys, which require an abundant supply of water to filter and purify the blood. Although the human need for water seems elementary, most people simply don't drink enough.

Alternative traditions consider water sacred to life. Their reverence for water appears in their recommendations on how much water should be drunk daily.

## *Ayurvedic Medicine and Water Therapy*

In Ayurveda, water is one of the five universal elements, out of which the doshas (body types) are formed. Pure water is essential to all the doshas. As a result, Ayurvedic physicians recommend the purest water possible. Ayurvedic yogis (holy men) have long preferred the Himalayas where they can drink from natural streams and springs of snowmelt. Today, Ayurveda advises people against drinking tap water that comes from water treatment plants until it has been purified with an appropriate home system. Tap water can contain large amounts of contaminates. Additives at the water plant often include chlorine and fluoride, both of which are toxic under conditions of time and dosage.

The correct amount depends on one's age and health conditions. To avoid an infection in the urinary tract and bladder, or to help treat such an infection, healthy young adults are advised to drink six to eight 8-ounce glasses a day. For those over fifty years of age, ten 8-ounce glasses a day is recommended. For people over sixty who are active and mobile, twelve 8-ounce glasses. People with kidney conditions should get the approval of their physician for the higher amounts.

Water is essential for cleansing and purification. The Sanskrit word for residual impurities in the body is *ama*. Ayurvedic physicians describe ama as a sticky substance that blocks normal channels of energy flow in the body. Ama can form obstructions in the veins and arteries, and the ducts that allow the flow of the metabolic compounds and enzymes within the body. It is a major blocker of biological energy, and a basic cause of chronic fatigue.

Here is an Ayurvedic purification method for removing *ama*, or residual impurities, from the body: Start with pure water, either distilled, or treated by charcoal filtration and reverse osmosis. Bring the water to a boil, and continue at a low boil for five to ten minutes. Pour the water into a thermos. During the day, sip the hot water at intervals as frequently as every half-hour. The quantity of water ingested is not as important as the frequency and temperature of the water, which is what creates the purifying effect.

## Traditional Chinese Medicine and Water Therapy

In Chinese medicine, essence refers to the vital fluids of the body. All living things are said to be born from fluid. The *I Ching, The Book of Change*, states that, "Heaven first produced water." The Taoist philosophy teaches that, "Water is the mother of the Three

Sources of Heaven, Earth, and Humans, and essence is the root of primal energy." The necessity for pure water is so important in Chinese medicine that Taoist teachers and physicians recommend the high mountains for the purity of mountain water. While there, some Taoists are said to have purged their systems of toxins by taking nothing but air and water for periods of time, a method known as "sniffing air and sipping dew." The objective of this method in traditional Chinese medicine is to detoxify the body, and to purify the body's water, which is considered the main ingredient in the body's vital essence.

Health counselors in traditional Chinese medicine advise against using tap water because it comes from water treatment plants. Public utility water has been shown to contain hundreds of contaminants, which can include aluminum, asbestos, benzene, cadmium, nitrates, pesticides, and polychlorinated biphenyls (PCBs.) Treatment plants frequently add chlorine and fluoride. Chlorine has been linked to heart and circulatory problems, and shown to kill off the helpful flora of the intestinal tract. Studies by the Argonne National Laboratories in the U.S. and the Nippon Dental University in Japan link fluoride with inducing and promoting cancer. To drink less than pure water is to go against the Taoist goals of health and longevity.

## Macrobiotics and Water

Macrobiotic cooks advise that careful attention be given to the amount of water used, as this changes the entire balance of the food. Along with the amount of water, the amount of oil, salt, and the fire used in cooking are important, as these are the ways in which vegetables and grains are turned into food, which in turn, makes the individual what he or she will become. As macrobiotic teacher Michio Kushi points out, "The best rice in the world cannot cure anyone unless it is prepared properly. Those who understand this know that simple dishes are the hardest to make; the highest art in cooking is the preparation of a bowl of rice."

## Western Medicine and Water

Until recently, Western science has downplayed the role of water in the maintenance of health, because the old scientific model stated that the solids (the *solute*) in the body were more important than the water (the *solvent*) in which they were dissolved. However, new research has demonstrated that the opposite is true, and water is the great sustainer of our minds and bodies. Health practitioners now look to water, rather than solids, as a primary method of maintaining optimum health.

Here are some of the roles that water plays in maintaining health:

- Water provides for essential cell function and volume. Any decrease in daily water intake affects the efficiency of cell activity.

- Water is the adhesive material that bonds together cell architecture.

- Water has an essential hydrolytic role in all aspects of body metabolism. Many chemical reactions (hydrolysis) are dependent on water, which is essential to the chemistry of life. Water transports oxygen to the cells.

- As water passes through cell membranes it creates hydro-electric energy, which is stored in energy pools that are the chemical sources of energy in the body.

- Water is a regulator of body functions. The solutions in which the enzymes, proteins, and hormones of the body are dissolved operate more efficiently when they are well-hydrated and have less viscosity.

- When the body is dehydrated, these solutions operate with less efficiency, and it may be at this point, a late stage of dehydration, that the thirst signal finally is felt.

### The Recommended Daily Dosage

Many nutritionists and physicians have increased their recommendations about how much water people need to drink each day. The current recommendation suggests that you drink six to eight

8-ounce glasses of water a day, which adds up to about two quarts of fluid intake for healthy adults. For active adults, as much as two and one-half quarts per day may be a better amount to assure proper hydration after sports.

The following drinks *do not* count toward your daily water intake:

- Alcohol is a diuretic (causes loss of fluids) and a urinary irritant.

- Coffee, colas, and caffeinated teas are diuretic and urinary irritants.

- Juices act as foods, rather than water, as they are a concentrated source of sugar.

- Milk is a protein food, rather than a way to restore fluids. Milk can stress the kidneys if they are not otherwise supplied with adequate amounts of pure water.

- Diet soft drinks are made with artificial sweeteners in addition to caffeine. The artificial sweetener aspartame is not recommended. As F. Batmanghelidj, M.D., points out "In the intestinal tract, aspartame converts to two highly excitatory neurotransmitters, as well as alcohol/formaldehyde—wood alcohol." People who consume diet soft drinks, he says, may experience weight gain, while those who consume optimum amounts of pure water will experience a loss of weight.

Drink these instead; they *do* count:

- Pure steam distilled or reverse osmosis treated water—all you want!

- Water with a small amount of juice in it.

- Non-caffeinated healthy herbal teas, hot or iced.

### Paying Attention to Water Quality

The quality of the water that you drink counts enormously. Most scientists now suggest that water be free of sodium and chlorine. Steam distilled and reverse osmosis treated water will meet this criterion.

Tap water does not. Do not drink tap water, which contains chlorine, fluoride, and a list of other chemicals and contaminants.

### Why Steam Distilled Water?

Steam distilled water is the most pure form of water you can get. The best steam distilling systems have a method of venting off all of the lighter-than-air gasses. As a final process, the water is filtered with a carbon filter. At the end of this process, distilled water has all the impurities and inorganic chemicals removed and is ready for immediate use by your body. Health practitioners call it free water because it does not have to be processed and purified by the kidneys and other organs, and is ready to go to work to hydrate your system.

> **REJECT FLUORIDE IN WATER SUPPLIES**
>
> The question of fluoridating water supplies by adding sodium fluoride at the treatment plant has been a public health controversy for some time. The alternative medicine approach is not to take sodium fluoride in your drinking water because it is unhealthful to your system.
>
> However, the use of fluoridated toothpaste can be helpful, as it acts against bacterial plaque, prevents tooth decay, and helps to protect gums. Periodontal health, the condition of the gums, is especially important in adults over forty. Parents should consult a dentist for the proper methods of protecting their children's teeth with fluoride, other than putting it in the drinking water.

Another good source is reverse osmosis treated water. This water is forced through a membrane, which removes unwanted contaminants. It is best used in combination with a charcoal filter. You can rent or buy an undersink unit for your home that will produce reverse osmosis water and charcoal filter it for use as cooking and drinking water.

### Chronic Pain and Dehydration

Health providers are now identifying dehydration as the cause of many health problems. In fact, some now believe chronic pain may be a possible indicator of dehydration. These chronic pains include: dyspeptic pain, rheumatoid arthritis pain, anginal pain (heart pain while walking, or even at rest), low back pain, intermittent leg pain on walking, migraine headaches, and colitis pain and its associated constipation. As F. Batmanghelidj, M.D. points out, water regulates all body functions, including the activity of the *solutes* it dissolves and circulates. For this reason, Dr. Batmanghelidj believes that many non-infectious recurring chronic pains result from the presence of toxins that are not removed by water.

If you have a chronic pain condition, it might be worthwhile for you to test this hypothesis. Begin by drinking an optimal amount of pure water for a period of several days to determine if the pain recedes. The amount of water to drink is approximately two to two and one-half quarts for healthy adults. During the water test, it is essential that the kidneys function properly to eliminate the extra water, and that urine output increases. Persons with kidney or urinary problems should consult a physician before testing for dehydration.

One chronic condition that has responded well to additional water is dyspeptic or digestive pain. This is because drinking a glass of water immediately passes into the intestines where it is absorbed into the body. Within thirty minutes a nearly identical amount of water is secreted into the stomach through the glandular layer of the mucosa, where it aids in the breakdown of foods in the stomach. The digestion of solid foods requires generous amounts of water.

Respiratory specialist physicians at the Vermont Lung Center also claim that if people with chronic bronchitis would drink ten glasses of pure water a day, their symptoms would be alleviated. This is because adequate amounts of water hydrate the lungs, bronchi, and the entire respiratory system, allowing its built-in defense systems to work as they are meant to do. Major surfaces of the respiratory system are coated with a layer of fluid, a mucous membrane, in which tiny hairs, called *cilia*, continually sweep debris and bacteria out of the body. This fluid layer is constantly losing water into the atmosphere. Replenishing this fluid by drinking lots of water keeps the system working.

### For Exercisers, Drink Before You're Thirsty

Many experts in exercise physiology believe that few athletes drink enough fluids before and during their activities to counter the ill

*"The simple truth is that water dehydration can cause disease. The solution for prevention and treatment of dehydration-produced diseases is water intake on a regular basis."*
—*F. Batmanghelidj, M.D.*

effects dehydration can have on performance and well-being. According to Jane Brody, noted nutritional author and columnist for the *New York Times,* thirst is an imprecise signal that often fails to kick in until the body is approaching the danger point. You may have already lost two quarts of water before thirst prompts you to start drinking. By the time you feel thirsty, your body is already dehydrated. The thirst signal is not a reliable way to know when it's time to drink more water. In fact, the thirst signal is the last outward sign of extreme dehydration.

**A WARNING FOR HIKERS AND MOUNTAIN BIKERS**

*One of the greatest rewards for staying energetic and fit is the ability to hike into wilderness areas where crystal clear streams and lakes abound. However, if you do, you must take precautions against the protozoan parasite Giardia lamblia. Giardia infection can cause upper abdominal pain, intestinal distress, and extreme weakness. It is spread by animals in the mountains, especially beavers. Be sure to buy a water filter pump to screen out the parasites and bacteria. Another alternative is to boil stream water or use iodine tablets to purify it.*

Water cools the body, so without water, the body temperature rises, as does the risk of heat exhaustion and heat stroke, which can be fatal. Without water, muscles also fatigue sooner and performance may decline by as much as 50 percent. The American College of Sports Medicine agreed in a recent position statement on exercise and fluid replacement that inadequate water intake leads to premature exhaustion. Instead of feeling relaxed and invigorated after a workout, the dehydrated exerciser is likely to feel stressed out, fatigued and lethargic, perhaps even headachy, dizzy, and nauseated.

Dr. Edward F. Coyle, director of the Human Performance Laboratory at the University of Texas at Austin, conducted an experiment with cyclists to show how dehydration hampers performance. He placed a group of cyclists in a heat chamber to dehydrate them and, before and after, had them peddle a bicycle ergometer that measured speed and heart rate. "When they saw how much dehydration slowed them down, it turned them into true believers about drinking more," the professor of kinesiology said.

If you sweat heavily, you are especially at risk and are least likely to drink enough. In fact, drinking water only replaces about two-thirds of the body water lost as sweat. It is common for individuals to dehydrate by 2 percent to 6 percent of their body weight during exercise in the heat. Some athletes believe that becoming acclimated to the heat helps the body conserve water. However, this is also erroneous because acclimatized individuals actually sweat more easily, so they need more water, not less, to avoid dehydration.

Physically active older people are also at an increased risk because their sense of thirst, sweat production, and the ability to concentrate urine declines with age. (Note: For this reason, it is especially dangerous to exercise in clothing that does not breathe in an effort to increase sweating and lose body fat.)

### Shower Water

Many people don't realize that chlorine and other vaporized chemicals present while showering and bathing can be harmful to your health. In fact, according to the Nader Report, one professor of chemistry at the University of Pittsburgh claims that exposure to vaporized chemicals in your shower and bath water is one hundred times greater than through drinking the same water. The reason for this is when chlorine and other chemicals are released into the air by the shower, you breathe them, and they are absorbed through your lungs. In addition, the warm water opens your pores, and your skin, the body's largest organ in surface area, absorbs the

---

**WATER RECOMMENDATIONS
FOR ATHLETES AND EXERCISERS**

*When you exercise, start out well hydrated. Ideally, drink about sixteen ounces of water about two hours before you exercise. Don't worry about the water; any excess will be lost through urination before you exercise. However, if you do not have to urinate within an hour, drink another eight ounces. If you cannot drink water two hours in advance, drink eight to sixteen ounces before starting your activity.*

*In either case, continue to drink water throughout your activity, consuming six to twelve ounces every fifteen to twenty minutes, especially if you are exercising in the heat. To increase the absorption of water into the blood, the water should be cool—from forty to fifty degrees Fahrenheit.*

*To be sure you have consumed enough water to prevent dehydration, weigh yourself before and after the activity. (If possible, weigh yourself unclothed, because sweaty clothes will skew the results). After exercising, note how much weight you have lost. For each pound of body weight loss, drink a pint (two cups) of water to replace the water you lost as sweat. Remember: don't judge by your thirst.*

chemicals into your system. A long, hot shower is especially harmful, as each doubling of shower time quadruples the amount of accumulating chemicals. Furthermore, the chlorine in shower water bonds with and destroys proteins in your hair, making it unmanageable and dry. Chlorinated water also contacts your eyes and large areas of your skin, which may become dry and itchy.

### THE CASE FOR SHOWER FILTERS

*Recent studies have confirmed that your risk for life-threatening diseases can increase when showering with chlorinated water. These risks include bladder and rectal cancer and heart disease. Small children, the elderly, and those with weakened immune systems are more susceptible. "Asthma, allergy, sinus, and emphysema sufferers should be aware that their conditions could become worse." Waterwise, Inc. 1995*

Fortunately there is a solution to this problem. To remove harmful chemicals from your shower or bath water, consider installing a water filter in place of your shower head. The filter contains a material, such as high purity copper and zinc alloy, that is designed to remove chlorine, lead, arsenic, hydrogen sulfide, nitrates, and several types of bacteria, including algae and fungi. The filters are designed to work well in warm or hot water. The benefits are immediately apparent, as the water and air become blessedly free of chlorine, your hair becomes silkier, and your skin smoother. You can also fill the tub through the shower filter for a chlorine-free bath.

Shower filters are available through health food stores, hardware or plumbing suppliers, or can be ordered by mail. Installation is usually simple, with no tools required. In the best of these filters, there is a replaceable cartridge that can be reversed for cleaning. Most filters last for about twenty thousand gallons of water, which for most people is about twelve to eighteen months.

## Chapter Recap

- You are 75 percent water and your brain is 85 percent water. Make it the right stuff!

- Do not drink tap water. The best water is pure water, made by steam distillation, or by reverse osmosis.

Both systems should be combined with a charcoal filter.

- In general, avoid sodium fluoride in your drinking water.

- Most people do not drink enough water. You need at least two quarts of pure water a day, about eight 8-ounce glasses. If you are active, you need closer to two and one-half quarts per day.

- Dehydration has been linked to many chronic conditions, including arthritis, back pain, migraines, and digestive problems.

- If you suffer from chronic conditions, you might try increasing the amount of water you drink to see if your pain is alleviated.

- Install a water filter in your shower and bath to avoid the dangers of inhaling chlorine and other vaporized chemicals from water while bathing.

*Recommended Reading*

Anselmo, Peter, with James S. Brooks, M.D. *Ayurvedic Secrets to Longevity and Health.* Englewood Cliffs, NJ: Prentice Hall, 1996.

Douillard, John. *Body, Mind and Sport, The Mind-Body Guide to Lifelong Fitness and Your Personal Best.* New York: Harmony Books, 1994.

Reid, Daniel. *The Complete Book of Chinese Health and Healing.* Boston: Shambala, 1995.

# Exercise—the Rejuvenator of Life

*I*n the last few decades, Western medicine has also come to realize that exercise is crucial to good health and longevity. Whereas Western science once thought aging was genetically programmed and inevitable, it has become clear in recent years that longevity is significantly promoted when people don't misuse, abuse, or neglect their body.

Most alternative healing traditions have always placed great stock in the importance of exercise to maintain vitality and lifelong health. Of course, many of these traditions have their roots in an era when people performed hard physical work in the fields or in cities, so it was only natural they had a high regard for keeping active to stay healthy. The idea of a sedentary lifestyle focused around a desk job, like many present day office workers, was unknown and unimaginable to them.

Despite this early necessity to perform daily physical labor, several alternative traditions, particularly the two systems of Ayurveda and Chinese medicine, evolved very precise ideas about how to keep the body and mind fit and healthy. In both of these traditions, exercise is perceived as a way to rejuvenate the vital life force (prana in the Ayurvedic tradition and chi in the Chinese

*93*

system). In line with this goal, each tradition developed a variety of exercises and physical movements that are intended to get stagnant vital energy flowing throughout the body. This chapter explores some of the most effective exercises from these traditions.

## Ayurvedic Fitness and Vitality

Ayurvedic fitness is founded on the combination of three elements: mental, emotional, and physical strength. Building all three simultaneously is a key principle in Ayurvedic exercise techniques.

Some of the main types of exercise used in Ayurveda are called *asanas*, meaning postures or positions. Many asanas may also be found in the discipline of yoga, but the application here is based on the health principles of Ayurveda. Asanas are designed to massage the body's inner organs, where the life force prana resides. This massaging action helps to stimulate the flow of blood and rejuvenate the life force, which energizes the body and keeps it healthy. Learning to practice asanas is not difficult. Some examples are given below.

### Warming Up—the Toning Up Postures

Before trying this exercise, note that Ayurvedic exercises should be avoided during pregnancy. People with health problems, especially those of a musculoskeletal nature, should consult a physician before beginning. Also, do not strain yourself to do the asanas. Over time your flexibility will increase. Do not force your body into any position. Wait three to four hours after eating a meal before starting the exercises. Allow thirty minutes after exercising before eating.

| EXERCISE | Toning Up, Posture A |
|---|---|

1. Sit comfortably on an exercise mat or folded blanket placed on the floor. Give yourself a gentle massage, starting at the top of your head and moving down to your toes. This will warm up the entire body, increase circulation, and prepare you for the exercises. Use a press-and-release

method of massage, pressing gently but firmly with both hands, and using both your palms and your fingers. Starting at the top of your head, work your way, inch by inch, down the head, neck, shoulders, and chest. This exercise should take from one to two minutes.

2. Massage your right arm, starting at the fingertips, moving up the top of the arm, then moving back down to the bottom of the arm. Repeat on the left arm.

3. Place your fingertips on your navel and palms on your abdomen. Press and release as you move up toward the heart.

4. Massage your lower back, moving toward the heart.

5. Starting with the toes, massage the right foot and leg, moving up until you reach the chest. Repeat with the left foot and leg up to the chest.

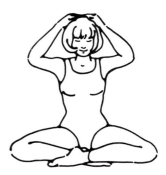

*Toning Up Posture A*

### Toning Up, Posture B *EXERCISE*

1. Lie on your back on the mat. Bring your knees to your chest, hug your knees, and roll slowly from side to side, allowing your head and neck to move freely. Roll from side to side five or six times.

2. Stretch out your arms and legs, lying quietly on your back. Close your eyes and relax. Get up slowly into the next position.

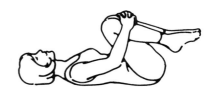

*Toning Up Posture B*

### The Seat-Firming Position *EXERCISE*

The seat-firming posture strengthens the legs, knees, ankles, and pelvic area. It is a good back exercise.

1. Kneel with your feet slightly apart. Move back toward a sitting position over your lower legs. If you have sufficient flexibility, sit on your feet, with your buttocks on your ankle area. Your back should be straight and your head held high.

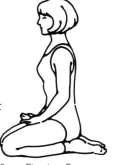

2. Rise to a kneeling position, back straight, shoulders relaxed. As you rise up, inhale.

3. Sit back again, toward your feet. As you sit back, exhale. Moving slowly, repeat rising up and sitting back twice. The exercise should take about thirty seconds.

*Seat Firming Posture*

EXERCISE                    *Head to Knee Position*

The head to knee position relaxes and stretches the back. It is a tonic for the abdominal organs and facilitates elimination.

1. Sit on the mat with your legs extended forward.

2. Keep the right leg straight, and bend your left leg, bringing the bottom of the left foot against the inside of the right thigh. Keep the left knee near the floor.

3. Lean forward, stretching your arms toward the right foot, touching the toes. At first your fingers may only reach to the lower leg or ankle. Bend the right leg slightly if necessary. Hold the position for ten to fifteen seconds and repeat, stretching again toward the right foot. Exhale as you stretch forward, and inhale as you straighten up.

4. Repeat this sequence, this time with your left leg straight and your right leg bent. Repeat twice, holding each time for ten to fifteen seconds. The exercise should take about one minute.

EXERCISE                    *The Rest Position*

At the completion of a round of exercises, the rest posture will refresh and invigorate you.

1. Lie on your back with legs extended and slightly apart.

2. Relax your arms at your sides, palms up.

3. Close your eyes, and lie quietly for a minute or two. Get up slowly.

## Yoga—Skill in Action

Yoga is a personal self-help system of health care and spiritual development. The word *yoga* means union or oneness and has been described as a systematic approach to becoming one with life.

There are different ways to practice yoga. One way is through postures, called *asanas,* aimed at toning the body and making it supple and flexible. This form of yoga is called *Hatha* (physical) yoga and has become widely known as yoga for health. Each posture has three purposes—bodily movement, mental control, and control of your breathing which can calm the body and mind. Yoga is both a mind and a body therapy, and the practice of some of the yoga postures is a way to achieve greater physical flexibility while at the same time achieve a greater sense of inner harmony and balance. The flexibility and other youthful characteristics developed through serious yoga practice can be maintained for life.

In active sports or strenuous exercises, you use up energy. In yoga classes, students report they feel tranquil after a class, yet have more energy. Slow and steady motion is the key to going into or coming out of postures. Hold a yoga pose for several seconds or even minutes and give attention to full, quiet breath. Your yoga instructor will encourage you to relax as the exercises are being done. Gently place your body into yoga postures. Done correctly, there's very little chance of injury or muscle stress. In performing yoga you should never strain, never go further than is comfortable. There is no hurry. Hurry and strain can retard your progress. A yoga session is designed for balance. You stretch to the right and then to the left. You bend back and then forward. You learn to recognize when one side is stronger and more flexible than the other. Thus harmony and balance are achieved with yoga practice.

People of all ages can practice yoga exercises. They are easily modified to meet your needs and physical condition. Don't be put off by the difficult looking postures you may see in a yoga book. A skilled teacher can adapt most asanas by using chairs, cushions, even a wall, or other props. A yoga practice can be tailor-made just for you. Yoga is a stress-free but powerful way to exercise. As with any exercise regimen, consult your health provider first.

*"If you can move your body one inch in any direction, you can do sufficient yoga to experience significant benefits almost at once."*
—*Richard Hittleman,*
Yoga for Health

*Warm Up Exercises*

Begin your exercises with a warm up routine. This can consist of up to a dozen easy-going postures. Here are two easy and classic warm-ups:

| E X E R C I S E | *The Standing Reach* |

The standing reach improves balance, expands the rib cage, and limbers the joints of the shoulders. Simply stand with your arms at your sides. To assist in keeping your balance, look at a spot on the wall in front of you. Breathe out completely through your nose.

1. As you breathe in, through your nose, bring your arms up in a circular movement from your sides to over your head. At the same time, lift yourself up on your toes.

2. The breath should be held for one second as you stretch toward the sky.

3. Exhale as you lower your arms to the sides, in the same circular movement, while lowering your feet until you are once again resting on your heels and toes. Repeat three times.

*The Standing Reach*

| E X E R C I S E | *The Complete Breath* |

The complete breath is an excellent way to visualize the inflow of prana or life force in a yoga exercise. Deep breathing also aids in relaxation, stress reduction, oxygenation of the blood, healing from respiratory problems, and an increase in the vital capacity of the lungs.

1. Start in a standing position with your arms relaxed at your sides. As you breathe out, pull in on your abdominal muscles to exhale completely. Let your muscles and neck go limp. For a moment, experience the depleted state when the life force and prana of the breath are absent. It is a time of minimum vitality.

2. As you inhale slowly through your nose, fill your lungs from the bottom up by pushing out your abdominal muscles. At the same time, raise your hands from your sides. Feel and visualize the rebirth of energy as the prana returns.

3. As your hands clasp over your head you have completed the breath, and your lungs are fully expanded. Visualize the peak of life force in your body.

4. Begin a slow exhalation as you lower your arms to your sides. Repeat this exercise three times.

When you are warmed up and ready to try an exercise posture, there is a variety from which to select.

| *The T Pose (Virabhadrasan)* | E X E R C I S E |
|---|---|

This exercise, called the T Pose, is intended to tone the legs, back, abdominal muscles, and abdominal organs. Other benefits can be a reduction in overall anxiety and a strengthened nervous system.

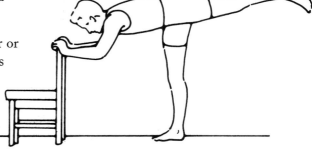

The T Pose

1. Support your hands on the back of a chair or railing and lean forward until your chest is parallel to the ground. Lift each leg into the parallel position several times to warm up. Raise one leg, keeping both knees straight. Focus on a spot on the ground to help retain your balance.

2. Gently release your hold on the railing and balance on one leg. Bring both hands together and point them at the ground. Hold for three seconds, then relax. Now do the same exercise with the other leg.

3. An alternate way to start this exercise, without the railing, is to lean your body forward with your hands supported on one knee. Raise the free leg to the parallel position. When you are in balance, bring your hands together and point

them at the floor. Hold for three seconds. Relax. Repeat
with the other leg. Except for the warm-up exercises, yoga
asanas should not be repeated more than three times. A
routine should be done once each day. A good yoga teacher
can be your guide into a lifetime of healthful mind/body
exercise.

## Chinese Exercises for the Control of Energy—Chi Gong

Chi gong, which is pronounced *chi-gung*, and may be spelled chi
kung, depending on the translator, is the Chinese skill of energy
control. Chi is the word for energy, as well as for breath and
air. Gong refers to skill or work. The combination of the two
means the energy work or energy skill we use to control our own
energy. Exercises, combined with conscious breathing, are integral to the practice of chi gong, and have been from very early
times in China. In the second century A.D. the scholar Cheng
Yuan-lin wrote, "Breathing practiced together with movements
resembling a bird, bear, and other animals helps move our chi,
nourishes our bodies, and builds our spirits." The four main
applications of chi gong are spiritual enlightenment, martial
power, health, and longevity. The primary benefits are balance and
harmony.

### Chi Gong Breathing and Movement Exercises

The following chi gong exercise is translated as "palms raised
to heaven to regulate the triple burners," which is intended to
enhance immunity and healing. In the Chinese organ-energy
system, the three burners are associated with the thorax, abdomen, and pelvis. This exercise is derived from *The Tendon
Changing Classic (Yi Jin Jing)* credited to the fifth century A.D.
Indian monk Bodhidharma, whom the Chinese called Ta Mo.
He brought the breathing exercises, called *pranayama,* from
India, and combined them with Chinese exercises into the
system of breathing and exercise that has become known as
chi gong.

This exercise begins in the horse stance, which is often used as the starting posture in chi gong exercises. It is an erect, standing posture, conducive to the flow of energy from the sacrum up along the spine to the head. This is a time to become tranquil in mind, relaxed in the body, and regulated in breath.

1. Slowly raise your hands along the pelvis, abdomen, and chest, while breathing in slowly and deeply. As you do so, contract slightly on the anus and pull in the abdominal muscles to place pressure on the internal organs.

2. When your hands reach your face, and you have taken in a full breath, turn the palms up and raise them above your head.

3. Keep extending the arms up until fully extended, with palms raised to heaven. Retain the breath for a moment.

4. Now relax and exhale slowly as you bring your arms down in a circular movement. As soon as you have your arms back in the horse stance you are ready to begin once more. Move through the exercise slowly and gracefully, observing the positions, and do twelve or more repetitions.

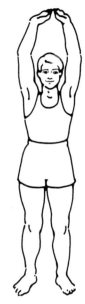

*Palms Raised to Heaven*

The chi gong teachers credit this exercise with regulating and balancing the upper burner (circulation and breathing); the middle burner (digestive organs and functions); and the lower burner (organs of elimination and sex). By energizing and stimulating the energies of these organ systems, it enhances their ability to function efficiently.

## The New Western Approach to Exercise

Western medicine has largely neglected physical exercise and nutrition in its understanding of good health and longevity. Even today, most Western doctors are not trained to teach their patients about the specific benefits of physical exercise or even which routines to use to lose weight, tone the body, or develop muscular strength. Indeed, those doctors who wanted to specialize in these areas were formerly shunted off into back offices, until some of them banded together to form their own clinics where they could effectively practice what became known as "sports medicine."

Today, there is a cadre of Western doctors who are leading the way to show the importance of exercise for everyone, regardless of age, prior exercise background, or health condition. It is generally believed that it is never too late to begin an exercise program and to derive benefits from it.

Over the past few decades, the emphasis in fitness training has been upon cardiovascular training, also known as aerobic fitness, to build heart and lung endurance. Aerobic fitness was popularized by Dr. Kenneth H. Cooper who focused on activities like running and cycling to derive impressive health benefits, especially for the heart and circulatory system.

However, the latest interpretation of fitness has shifted toward a balance of four components.

- *Cardiorespiratory endurance*—measured in the sustained ability of the heart, lungs, and blood vessels to deliver oxygen to your body's cells.

- *Muscular fitness*—both muscular strength—the force a muscle produces in one effort—and muscular endurance—the ability to repeat that force in rapid succession.

- *Body flexibility*—the ability of your joints to move freely through their full range of motion without discomfort or pain.

- *Body lean mass composition*—a measure of how much of your body mass is lean muscle and bone, as compared to how much is fat.

Each component contributes to your health and potential for a long life by reducing the risk of getting chronic muscular and joint ailments that many people get as they age. Lifestyle diseases that result from a weak heart, a poor circulatory system, or from being overweight are also limited. In other words, if you work on meeting the standards of all four components for your age category and lifestyle, you can significantly improve your chances of a long, healthy life.

*Evaluating Your Current Fitness in the Four Areas*
To plan an appropriate fitness program for yourself, you should begin by finding out where you stand on the four components of fitness. Each component has a specific test that is used to measure an individual's current physical condition. Some sports institutes perform these tests using sophisticated equipment which operate at a high cost. There are, however, simple, inexpensive home tests you can do on your own, which are explained on the following pages.

**NOTE**

*Before taking any tests, it is wise to inform your health provider that you intend to initiate a physical fitness program. He or she can then counsel you on any risks you might be subject to, depending on your current health condition, family history, and other factors. If you are a man over forty or a woman over fifty, or if you have any indications of heart disease, you should consult a physician first.*

*Evaluate Your Cardiorespiratory Endurance*                          **E X E R C I S E**

A number of simple tests, such as the Rockport Fitness Walking Test, developed for the Rockport Walking Institute, can be used to measure cardiorespiratory health. In the Rockport test you walk a measured mile, noting the time it takes and your pulse rate when finished.

1. Do not eat, drink coffee or tea, or smoke for at least two hours before beginning. Warm up by walking slowly until your limbs feel warm.

2. Count your pulse rate. Multiply it times the number of minutes it took to complete the walk. (This number will be higher than the rate your heart was actually beating during the walk.)

3. Evaluate. The Rockport test suggests that men and women in peak condition should have a heartbeat count of 2,000 or lower. Those in relatively poor shape may have a count as high as 3,500. Even if your heart rate is at the lower end of this range, there is room for improvement.

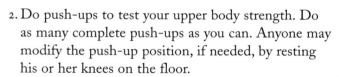

| E X E R C I S E | *Muscular Fitness* |

Test your strength. Start with an aerobic warm-up for ten minutes, until you feel warm and your heart rate gradually increases. Try these simple tests used by the University of California at Berkeley. (Avoid any undue strain on your neck.)

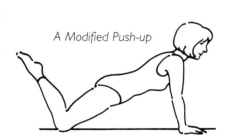

*The Abdominal Hold*

*A Modified Push-up*

1. Do an abdominal hold to evaluate middle body strength. Lie on the floor with your knees raised comfortably. With your hands behind your head, raise your upper body to a forty-five degree angle from the floor and hold as long as you can.

2. Do push-ups to test your upper body strength. Do as many complete push-ups as you can. Anyone may modify the push-up position, if needed, by resting his or her knees on the floor.

3. Do a wall sit to test your quadriceps. Put your back against a wall, and bend your knees, and slide your torso down until your hip joints are level with your knees. (Your lower legs should be at a right angle to your thighs.) Hold.

4. Check the ratings in the charts to measure your strength. These numbers are for men in their twenties. Decrease ratings by 15 percent for every 10 years of increasing age. Values for women are on average approximately 20 to 25 percent less than for men.

*The Wall Sit*

FITNESS LEVELS

| | Wall Sit | Abdominal Hold | Push Ups |
|---|---|---|---|
| *High* | 90 seconds | 25 seconds | 25 repetitions |
| *Average* | 60 seconds | 15 seconds | 15 repetitions |
| *Below Average* | 30 seconds | 5 seconds | 5 repetitions |
| *Low* | less than 30 seconds | less than 5 seconds | less than 5 repetitions |

## Body Mass Composition

EXERCISE

Federal health authorities now consider a body mass of 25 or more to be overweight (previously the number was 27). The following formula will give you an approximate idea of your body mass.

1. Multiply your weight by 703.

2. Square your height, that is, multiply height in inches by height in inches.

3. Divide the answer in step one by the answer in step two. The result is your body mass.

## Building Your Fitness

Here's how you can improve your fitness in each of the four areas.

### Cardiovascular Fitness Program

The amount of aerobic exercise that you need, according to the American College of Sports Medicine, is twenty to sixty minutes, three times a week, at 60 percent of your maximum heart rate capacity. A person's maximum heart rate capacity is measured in heartbeats per minute based on one's age. Use the following chart to look up your capacity.

According to fitness specialist Robert Arnott, M.D., the 100 percent figure is hard to achieve and impossible to maintain, 90 percent is for top athletes in competition, 80 percent can be done

### MAXIMUM HEART RATE ACCORDING TO AGE

|      | 20s | 30s | 40s | 50s | 60s | 70s | 80s | 90s | 100 |
|------|-----|-----|-----|-----|-----|-----|-----|-----|-----|
| 100% | 200 | 190 | 180 | 170 | 160 | 150 | 140 | 130 | 120 |
| 90%  | 180 | 171 | 162 | 153 | 144 | 135 | 126 | 117 | 108 |
| 80%  | 160 | 152 | 144 | 136 | 128 | 120 | 112 | 104 | 96  |
| 70%  | 140 | 133 | 126 | 119 | 112 | 105 | 98  | 91  | 84  |
| 60%  | 120 | 114 | 108 | 102 | 96  | 90  | 84  | 78  | 72  |
| 50%  | 100 | 95  | 90  | 85  | 80  | 75  |     |     |     |
| 40%  | 80  | 76  | 72  |     |     |     |     |     |     |

one or two days a week by someone in really good condition, 70 percent is the practical top end for general fitness, 60 percent is what you need for a good workout, and below 50 percent you are coasting.

### Muscular Strength and Endurance Fitness Program

There are three basic methods by which you can build your muscular strength and endurance: free weights, exercise machines, and good old-fashioned muscle exercises. The following chart compares the three methods.

If you are adverse to free weights or joining a club to use machines, it can be well worth your effort to try exercising on your own. Most muscular exercises are not complicated and can be learned quickly. Here are two examples among many you can find in exercise books. If you have any questions, or any difficulty performing the exercises, check with a fitness trainer for specific advice.

### Abdominal Muscle Strengthening Exercise

We all use the abdominal muscles constantly. They power or stabilize the body in almost every kind of exercise, helping to transfer forces between the upper and lower body. If you want a strong back and good posture, work on the abs. Think of them as very

BUILDING MUSCLE STRENGTH

| | *Advantages* | *Disadvantages* |
|---|---|---|
| *Free weights* | Free weights are versatile, allowing you to work many muscle groups. They are relatively inexpensive, and can improve your coordination and balance. One exercise with free weights can work a number of different muscle groups at the same time. | Free weights can cause injury if they are dropped or slip on you. It can be time consuming to adjust and change free weights. |
| *Machines* | Exercise machines, like Nautilus and others, are easy to use and relatively safe. They can isolate muscle groups and place demand on them through the full range of motion. | The best machines are expensive and take up space in your home. Joining a club to use exercise machines can be expensive. |
| *Exercise* | Once they have been properly learned, exercises require little equipment or expense, and can be performed at the time and place that work best for you. A wide range of muscle groups can be exercised. | Exercises performed improperly can subject parts of the body to undue stress. Proper instruction and monitoring are available, and should be used until you are doing the exercise correctly. |

powerful rubber bands that act as a natural girdle, supporting and protecting the internal organs and the muscles of the back. The shape of your abdominal muscles also affects your appearance. The *rectus abdominis* muscle is the principal mover of the spine when you bend forward. It's also the muscle that gives the washboard appearance to well-developed abdomens.

To strengthen and tone the abdominal muscles, try this elegant exercise with a prosaic name: the crunch. The crunch is a more efficient exercise than the traditional sit-up to condition the abdominal muscles, as it emphasizes the important layer of muscle that covers your midsection from the pubic bone to the rib cage. When performed correctly, the crunch allows both men and women to strengthen their abdominal muscles without stressing the small of the back or the muscles of the neck.

*The Crunch*

EXERCISE                                    *The Crunch*

1. Place an exercise mat or padding on the floor under your back and head. Lie with your back flat on the floor and your legs drawn up to about a ninety-degree angle. (See the illustrations.)

2. Support the back of your neck just below your head with your hands. Point your elbows forward and up. Slowly lift the upper body with your abdominal muscles, raising yourself off the mat no higher than the bottom of your shoulder blades. Exhale during exertion. Breathe in to your upper chest in rapid puffs when the work grows intense.

3. Let the weight of your head hang back, supported by your hands.

4. Roll back down as slowly as possible, using your abdominal muscles to resist the force of gravity. This also helps protect against back strain.

To customize the crunch to your ability level, you can perform it with different arm positions: arms forward for least effort, arms crossed over the chest for more exertion, elbows out, hands behind head for even more effort.

*Basic Crunch Position with Modified Arm Positions*

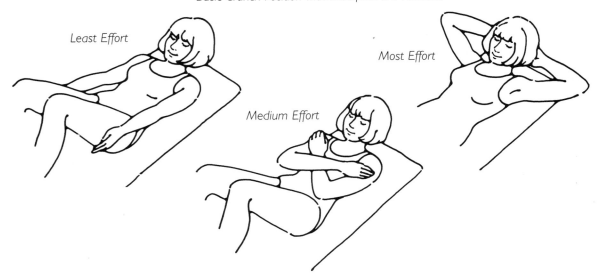

*Least Effort*

*Most Effort*

*Medium Effort*

## Back Strengthening—The Pelvic Tilt

EXE 1

To strengthen the back, look to the muscles in the erector spinae group. These run along both sides of the spine, from the base of the spine to the chest. They are extremely important in the maintenance of good posture and a pain-free back.

Here is a simple but effective exercise to strengthen the back.

1. Lie on the floor with a mat under your head and hips. Place your hands under your head.

2. Bend your legs up and rest your feet flat on the floor. Flatten your lower back.

3. Slowly roll the hips up until your waistline lifts off the floor. Feel your lower spine lengthen as the pelvis tilts. Hold for ten seconds, then slowly roll back down. Repeat three times.

*The Pelvic Tilt*

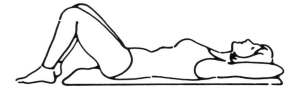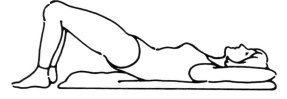

## Body Flexibility Fitness Program

EXERCISE

If you have been stretching to warm up for exercise or sports, listen up. A lot of people who go through a stretching routine to avoid injury wind up being injured by the stretches themselves. At the very least, you should warm up before stretching.

Training your muscles to stretch is a lot like training them for strength. Here are the top tips for doing it successfully.

1. Allow time after eating before serious stretching.

2. Warm up with a five to ten minute aerobic exercise until you begin to sweat.

3. Never force a stretch.

4. Remain relaxed and breathe slowly and fully. Exhale as you go into a stretch.

5. Work the parts of the body that need more flexibility.

6. When stretching one side of the body, be sure to do the same stretches on the other side.

7. Work at your own pace.

8. Do not stretch torn or sore muscles.

9. To build and maintain gains in your flexibility, continue stretching about three times a week.

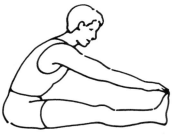

*Test Your Flexibility*

---

EXERCISE                                    *Stretches*

The elongation stretch should be used before every stretching session.

1. Lie on the floor or on a mat, face up.

2. Stretch your arms out above your head, keeping them flat along the floor. Through the entire stretch, breathe deeply and slowly.

3. Bring your legs together, flat on the floor.

4. Extend your legs and arms as far as you can, pointing your toes and fingers away from you. Turn the palms of your hands toward the ceiling.

5. Tilt your pelvis downward to gradually extend the curve of your back.

6. Tuck in your chin.

7. Hold the position for approximately ten seconds, then relax. Repeat the elongation stretch three times. This is a full body stretch and can be felt in the lower back, upper back, shoulders, chest, sides, and abdominals, as well as in your arms and legs.

*Stretches to Avoid*

Fitness trainers have identified some stretches that most people should avoid because they place excessive stress on ligaments, muscles, and joints. These include:

- *Toe touching* with locked knees

- *The plow*—where all the weight is on the back of the neck

- *Leg kicks* with the knee locked

- *The hurdler's stretch*

## Body Composition Program

The goal of a body composition modification program is to reduce the percentage of fat in your body while adding muscle. Many people are confused by the fact that adding muscle actually increases your weight because muscle is denser than fat. A pound of muscle takes up about 20 percent less space than a pound of fat.

However, while your weight may increase, you should not mind because the added muscle will tone and compact your body, making it appear you have lost weight. Measurements, like your waistline, will often reduce as you lose fat and add muscle. Many exercises can help you lose fat while adding muscle. The key to losing fat is to burn calories.

The chart on page 112 shows you how many calories are burned in eight different types of activities.

*Getting Motivated to Exercise*

Most of us have difficulty getting motivated to start and maintain a serious and consistent fitness program. Life often does not seem to afford us the time to exercise the recommended three times per week for thirty minutes. However, if you want to stay healthy and increase your longevity, you have to recognize that fitness is as important as nutrition in preventing the onset of illness and in slowing down the biological clock. Exercise will allow you to act and feel younger than your chronological age.

CALORIES BURNED IN 50 MINUTES

| Activity | Calories Burned |
|---|---|
| Walking | 2.5 mph - 105<br>4.5 mph - 200<br>6.0 mph - 370 |
| Cycling | 5.5 mph - 130<br>10 mph - 220<br>13 mph - 320 |
| Rowing | Light: 200<br>Vigorous: 420 |
| Skiing | Downhill: 300<br>Cross Country: 200 - 560 |
| Racquet Sports | Badminton: 175<br>Tennis: 210<br>Racquetball: 360<br>Squash: 420 |
| Aerobic Dance | Light: 120<br>Moderate: 200<br>Vigorous: 300 |
| Running | 5.5 mph 320<br>7.5 mph 430<br>10 mph 550 |
| Swimming | 25 yds/minute: 180<br>40 yds/minute: 260<br>50 yds/minute: 375 |

*These calorie expenditures are based on a person weighing 150 lbs. For every 15 lbs. over that weight add 10 percent. Subtract 10 percent for every 15 lbs. under that weight.*

One way to help a negative attitude about finding the time to exercise is to reframe your thinking so that you can train smart. Training smart means training more efficiently, and improving more rapidly, given the time you are able to allocate to fitness training. By training smart you will gain many benefits. You will increase your speed and endurance. You will become efficient in the use of your training time. You will avoid injury, and as a final bonus, you will stay forever younger than the date on your birth certificate says you are.

So, how do you train smart? The answer, according to Dr. Robert Arnott is to think of yourself as an athlete. This is called a paradigm shift, a new way of seeing an issue. Rather than thinking of yourself as an inexperienced or half-hearted person who occasionally exercises, make a leap to a new way of seeing your lifelong fitness. Let go of the conventional idea that you are inevitably going to spend the rest of your life with declining abilities.

> ### THE MYTH OF "MAINTENANCE FREE" LIVING
>
> *In his book, Dr. Bob Arnott's* Guide to Turning Back the Clock, *Robert Arnott states that our twenties are the last decade of maintenance free living. He points out that beginning at age forty, a sedentary male will lose six pounds of muscle, nearly 7 percent of heart function, and 8 percent of lung function every ten years. To illustrate the impact that such loss can have, consider what thigh muscles look like at age twenty and at age seventy.*
>
> *Fortunately, exercise can help slow down the aging process. By exercising and working on all four components of a fitness program, you can decelerate the rate at which you lose heart and lung function, and avoid losing muscle tone nearly completely.*

To be an athlete is to be physically strong and active. If you are in your twenties and not exercising, this should be relatively easy to do, as you can still function at your physical best with only a small amount of training and effort. If you are in your thirties, forties, or fifties and have not been exercising consistently, you will clearly need to focus your efforts on changing these unhealthy habits.

One fun idea to help increase your motivation is to take a photo of yourself—just as you are—and scan it into your computer (or borrow a friend's computer and scanner). Then, using image viewing and software, modify the photo so that you take on a healthier, more toned-up appearance. Then print out this new image of yourself and hang it on your wall as a motivator that helps you strive for a new future.

However, don't let your external appearance be the sole force driving your motivation. The strongest motivation actually comes from inside you, from your own increasing sense of self and your own wisdom about what it takes to be truly healthy. Make exercise a part of life because you are confident it will improve your health and extend your life.

### *A Fitness Summary*

You have a choice in how you approach fitness. It doesn't need to be a test of courage and dedication. Fitness can be fun. There are many activities you can choose from based on your interests, abilities, and time. Keep in mind that many types of activities improve more than one component of your fitness. Here are some possibilities:

- *Cardiorespiratory conditioning*—The ability of the heart and lungs to function efficiently is enhanced by activities that sustain a raised heart rate for at least twenty consecutive minutes without making you become breathless. You can choose from: brisk walking or jogging, swimming laps, cycling, skating, cross-country skiing, step aerobics, water aerobics, jumping rope, playing vigorous tennis, squash or racquetball, and working out on a treadmill, ski machine, or exercise bicycle.

- *Muscular strength and endurance*—Muscles must be stressed to get stronger. Activities that promote muscular strength and endurance may also promote cardiorespiratory conditioning. Be careful though, working on only certain muscle groups can cause other opposing muscles to become relatively neglected, which increases the risk of injury. It is always wise to aim for balance. For example, people who walk or jog often neglect their upper body strength. To avoid this condition, try lifting free weights, swimming the crawl, or using a rowing machine.

- *Flexibility*—Avoid injury to your body by making sure your muscles and joints can move freely through their full range of motion. Be careful as exercises that promote endurance or strength may tighten other muscle groups. For instance, runners often improve the muscles in the back of their legs, but in doing so, they increase their vulnerability to knee and ankle injuries. It is best to offset muscle conditioning by doing exercises to promote flexibility all over the body. These include gentle, nonstressful stretching activities of your choice. Be sure to warm up your muscles before you stretch, and stretch again after exercising.

- *Reducing body fat—* Burning calories is essential to losing body fat and increasing the ratio of muscle to fat. The biggest calorie burners are the activities that require the sustained use of large muscle groups in the legs, arms, and torso.

**SEE YOUR DOCTOR**

*The American College of Sports Medicine recommends that healthy men over age forty and women over age fifty who wish to start a vigorous exercise program should first consult a physician. Others should see a physician if they have two or more risk factors or symptoms for heart disease. These include recurrent chest pain, high blood pressure or high cholesterol levels, smoking, or obesity. Regardless of your age, you should also consult a physician if you have any cardiovascular, lung, or joint-muscle conditions.*

*The Good News—Sex Can Also Be Rejuvenating*

Most of us don't think of sex as a form of preventive health, but many ancient healing traditions view sex as rejuvenating. In Chinese medicine, sexual vitality is believed to demonstrate strong protective powers of immunity and resistance to disease. It is thought that sexual discipline conserves and enhances energy, allowing the transformation of sexual energy into spiritual vitality. Aging may be caused by the absence of reproductive activity. By continuing sexual intercourse into later life, it is felt, sexual vitality will be enhanced, perhaps restraining the genetic message which tells the body to age.

The significance of this should not be taken lightly. Couples may forego sex because they are tired or too stressed, without realizing that sex, like exercise, can actually reduce their stress, and make them feel better. After all, sex increases the heart and breathing rate (the aerobic component), works an assortment of muscle groups, and can also provide muscle stretching for flexibility.

In traditional Chinese medicine, it is thought that excessive or undisciplined sexual activity drains the body of vital nutrients from other body systems. Men are depleted of kidney energy due to excessive ejaculation, and women are depleted of kidney energy due to insufficient or incomplete orgasm. The Chinese medicine theory is that the body seeks to maintain reproductive sexual potency at all costs, to preserve and propagate the species. Vital nutrients needed in other systems of the body will be borrowed, if necessary, to protect the reproductive system. Therefore, if sexual vitality is diminished, it is an indicator that the entire system is depleted and in need of restoration. One solution is found in the Tao of Yin and Yang. Yin is satisfied in women through orgasm, while yang in men is controlled by the discipline of regulating ejaculation to prevent exhaustion. The disciplines are modified to reflect the age and health of the persons. Traditional Chinese medicine teaches that sex is an efficient and effective way to enhance immunity, increase energy, extend life, and build up abundant supplies of hormone essence.

---

**EXERCISE AND ROMANCE—AN UNBEATABLE COMBINATION**

*A Club Med™ survey of couples on vacation revealed some interesting results that point to a form of synergy which partners can develop if they exercise together in moderation.*

- *Vacationing couples who played tennis against each other were three times more likely to have romantic moments than those couples who played on the same side.*

- *Of the Club Med™ couples who went horseback riding, 75 percent held hands more than usual, and 71 percent kissed more.*

- *Dieting couples were three times as likely to argue as those who were not watching their weight.*

- *And 49 percent of the couples who enjoyed scuba diving found their partners became more complimentary afterward.*

---

## Chapter Recap

- Ayurvedic asanas, or positions, are based on the concept of massaging the inner organs and stimulating the circulatory system.

- Yoga exercises can reduce stress and increase flexibility.

- The Chinese martial art of chi gong is based on revitalizing your energy by moving your chi throughout your body.

- A growing cadre of Western physicians is showing the important role physical fitness plays in preventive medicine.

- Physical fitness is divided into four components: cardiorespiratory (heart & lung) endurance, muscle strength, flexibility, and body composition. By working on all four components through a consistent program of exercises and athletics of your choice, you can significantly improve your fitness, increase your resistance to disease, and increase your longevity by avoiding degenerative diseases. You really can turn back your biological clock by becoming an athlete.

*Recommended Reading*

Douillard, John. *Body, Mind and Sport* New York: Harmony Books, 1994.

Eisenberg, David M.D. with Thomas Lee Wright. *Encounters with Qi, Exploring Chinese Medicine.* New York: W.W. Norton & Company, 1985.

White, Timothy P. Ph.D. and the editors of the University of California at Berkeley Wellness Letter, *The Wellness Guide to Lifelong Fitness,* New York: Rebus distributed by Random House, 1993.

# *Air — the Breath of Life*

*T*he air you breathe is your most immediate and vital source of health. This source is often overlooked because breathing is an automatic process that goes on unconsciously day and night, without your conscious awareness. This chapter will increase your awareness of your breathing, and introduce you to a variety of exercises that will relax you and empower you to feel healthier. You will understand the role of proper breathing in health, healing, and cardiovascular fitness, and how burning oxygen efficiently will literally light up your life.

The great natural healing systems of the world, such as Ayurveda, yoga, Chinese medicine, and mind/body medicine all insist on conscious control of breath. Their focus on conscious control is not accidental; rather these traditions all consider breathing to be sacred to life itself. You will learn some of the techniques of these traditions to increase the conscious control of your breath, as well as learn the techniques of abdominal breathing developed by Western medicine. Let this be an introduction to your most vital health resource, one that you, your body, and your brain need to have in top shape every minute of every day.

IN THIS CHAPTER:

- *The Ayurvedic view of the importance of walking and meditation*

- *Chinese chi gong exercises to revitalize your chi*

- *The yoga discipline of breath control*

- *Meditation and tranquility breathing*

- *Deep diaphragmatic breathing—Western style*

- *Aerobics and deep breathing*

## Ayurvedic Medicine, Air, and Breathing

Ayurveda is perhaps the oldest tradition to recognize the importance of clean, pure air in the maintenance of health, despite the fact that thousands of years ago, the chemistry of air was unknown. Ayurveda held the breath sacred. It is thus not surprising that the Ayurvedic term for breathing is prana. In the Ayurvedic tradition, air is also one of the five primary elements of the universe.

Modern science has learned a great deal about the elegant design of the human respiratory system. When we breathe in, air enters the nasal cavity, where the air is filtered and warmed. Contaminant particles that might be in the air, such as pollen or soot, are accelerated in the air stream by breathing, and forced to make a sharp turn in a nasal passage. The air makes the turn, but most of the unwanted particles strike a surface covered with moisture where they are captured, and later swept out of the nasal cavity by the action of the cilia, tiny hairs that beat rhythmically. This is but one example of the body's protective system, which can handle just about any environmental threat except tobacco smoke, which paralyzes the cilia for approximately twenty minutes after smoking. While in the nasal cavity, the air also supplies information to the brain by way of the olfactory nerve, the sense of smell, which transports signals to the brain.

Ayurvedic health counselors teach that the body's life force is carried into the body by breathing oxygen. As a result, knowledge and control of one's breath is the key to optimum physical and mental performance. (This is why breathing exercises are part of Ayurvedic medicine.) Ayurvedic physicians recommend fresh air walks twice a day. People who follow this practice are supposed to see an immediate increase in their sense of well-being and vitality.

To increase one's focus on conscious breathing, Ayurveda also teaches specific breathing meditation exercises. Here is an example of one simple exercise:

EXERCISE                              *Ayurvedic Breathing*

1. Sit in a straight-backed chair, or on a mat on the floor.

2. Start by breathing normally. Gradually direct your attention toward your breathing. Become aware of the inflow and outflow of your breath, without trying to control it.

3. Neither resist nor encourage your breath, allow it to stabilize into its own rhythm.

4. If you become distracted by your thoughts, don't resist, and don't let it bother you. Simply let your awareness return to your breathing.

5. Do the breathing meditation for fifteen minutes, then allow two or three minutes for your awareness to return to the world around you.

6. Do the breathing meditation in the morning and evening of every day. The benefits you receive will be relaxation, reduction of stress, and restoration of energy.

### The Yoga Discipline of Breath Control

In the yoga discipline, breathing exercises are called *pranayama*, which means control of prana. The purpose of pranayama is to purify the body. When you exhale, impurities from the body are removed through the lungs; when you inhale, you inhale not only oxygen, but also universal energy and knowledge.

### Traditional Chinese Medicine and Breathing Exercise

In the Chinese medical view, healthful breathing comes from slow, easy, rhythmic exercises done on a daily basis. These breathing exercises promote the circulation of one's vital essence, *chi*, throughout the body. Chinese medicine also believes that deep breathing causes the body to switch from its normal functioning to a rejuvenating function with enhanced disease resistance and improved circulation of the blood. Western scientists have also discovered that slow breathing exercises can cause the body to switch from the sympathetic nervous system to the parasympathetic branch of the autonomous nervous system. This enhances the positive biofeedback between the endocrine and nervous systems, thus helping the immune system. The Taoist physician Sun Ssumo, in the seventh century A.D., pointed out the benefits of correct, deep breathing in his medical book, *Precious Recipes*, "When correct breathing is practiced, myriad ailments will not occur. When breathing is depressed or strained, all sorts of diseases will arise. Those who wish to nurture their lives must first learn the correct method of controlling breath and balancing energy. These breathing exercises can cure all ailments great and small."

One of the most important types of breathing exercises developed in Chinese medicine is known as *chi gong* (also spelled Qigong), which literally means energy work. As mentioned earlier, chi gong is a Chinese exercise discipline which has the purposes of martial arts skill, spiritual enlightenment, health, and long life. Chi gong emphasizes gentle, soft exercises and deep breathing and is based on moving one's yin and yang energies around. Yin and yang are complementary poles of the same basic energy. When inhaling we are in the yin polarity, accumulating and concentrating air into the body. When exhaling, we are in the yang polarity, releasing and expanding air out of the body. In this way, chi gong helps balance the two energies in a gentle, smooth flow.

## *Meditation and Tranquility Breathing*

Meditation, which by definition includes slow, deep breathing to relax the mind and body, fostering tranquility and healing. It is an integral part of natural healing systems such as traditional Chinese medicine and Ayurveda, and now has an important role in Western mind/body medicine. These meditation techniques are based on a discipline of conscious controlled breathing, where deep, regular breathing allows the mind to become tranquil and receptive.

The goal of tranquility breathing is to allow you to take control over moods and emotions connected with your respiration rate. For example, fear and anger are associated with breathing that is shallow, rapid, and irregular. By using voluntary control over your breathing to make it slow, deep, and regular a change of emotional state called centeredness, follows.

Try the following tranquility breathing exercise.

| *Tranquility Breathing Exercise* | E X E R C I S E |
|---|---|

1. Place the tip of your tongue behind your upper front teeth. Purse your lips if this feels awkward. Inhale and exhale in this exercise with your tongue in that position. Follow these steps:

2. Exhale completely through your mouth. You will hear a whoosh sound as the air goes around your tongue.

3. Now close your mouth and inhale quietly through your nose to a mental count of four.

4. Hold your breath for a count of seven.

5. Exhale completely through your mouth to a count of eight; again, you will hear a whoosh sound as the air exhales.

This is one breath. Now inhale again and repeat the cycle three more times for a total of four breaths. Note that you always inhale *quietly* through your nose, and you exhale through your mouth with an audible whoosh sound. Note also, the ratio used in this exercise: four beats to inhale; seven beats hold; and eight beats to exhale. This ratio is very important. If you have trouble holding your breath for seven beats, you can speed up the exercise by counting faster for each step. Keep the ratio of 4:7:8. With practice, you will be able to slow your breath down and get used to inhaling and exhaling deeply.

The conscious control of breath is a natural tranquilizer for the nervous system. Medical experts say there is a bonus to these breathing techniques in that, unlike tranquilizing drugs which are often effective when you first take them but lose their power over time, tranquility breathing exercises gain in power with repetition and practice. Try the one described above at least twice a day, with no more than four breaths at one time for the first month of practice. Later you can extend it to eight breaths.

## *The Western Approach—Deep Abdominal Breathing*

In the West, deep breathing has been an art mostly reserved for actors, singers, and public speakers. However, deep breathing is now becoming popular among many people who recognize the health benefits that can be gained from its practice.

Perhaps the most popular form of deep breathing is known as abdominal or diaphragmatic breathing. In this form of exercise, the lungs are filled from the abdomen on up to the chest. This technique is often taught to singers and actors because it allows them greater control over their breath, and to inhale and exhale a greater volume of air. A typical daytime breath is about five hundred cubic centimeters of air, about half a pint. However, with deep, voluntary breathing, you can move eight to ten times more air.

> *"When the mind is calm and stable, the vitality of life circulates harmoniously throughout the body. If the body is nourished and protected by this circulation of vitality, how can it possibly become ill?"*
>
> —The Yellow Emperor's Classic of Internal Medicine, *China, second century BC*

| E X E R C I S E | *Deep Abdominal Breathing* |
| --- | --- |

1. Sit in a straight chair with your back straight but relaxed. If at any time you feel dizzy or light-headed during this exercise, simply resume normal breathing. It is best to breathe through your nose, which filters and warms the air.

2. Place your hands on your abdomen. Contract your abdominal muscles and exhale through your nose as much air as possible. While exhaling, you can feel your abdomen going in. Inhale slowly, letting your abdomen expand as though it is being filled with air. At this time only your abdomen is rising as the lower parts of your lungs fill with air. This is abdominal breathing. Try it a few more times.

3. On your next inhalation, allow the air to rise into your chest. You can feel your rib cage expand.

4. Continue to inhale, and you will feel the air rising to the upper part of your chest. When air inflates the top of your lungs you will feel your collarbone rise slightly. Be careful not to draw your abdomen in at this point.

5. To exhale, repeat the process in reverse, from top to bottom. Allow air to escape from the collarbone area, the chest, and finally from the abdomen, using your abdominal muscles to push out the remaining air.

6. You have now done a complete deep breathing exercise. Practice this technique daily, and the next time you take a breathing test you can amaze your doctor. What's more important, you will be supplying your body with the oxygen that it needs.

### Breathing While Exercising

The importance of effective breathing is a key element when doing aerobic exercise. Aerobic is a word derived from the Greek meaning with oxygen. Aerobic exercises include brisk walking, swimming, or distance running—all of which depend on a continuous supply of oxygen. In short, unless you can breathe deeply, it is difficult to do well with aerobic exercises.

In *The Wellness Guide to Lifelong Fitness*, Timothy P. White, Ph.D. and the editors of the *U.C. Berkeley Wellness Letter* write, "Of all the elements of fitness, the most crucial is that of cardiorespiratory endurance—the sustained ability of the heart, lungs, and blood vessels to take oxygen from the air and deliver it and other nutrients throughout the body to every cell." Conscious, efficient breathing is essential to athletic success, and the effect that breathing habits have in causing, preventing, or correcting health problems is equally dynamic.

## Chapter Recap

- The Ayurvedic tradition recommends two daily walks for clean pure air, as well as the practice of breathing exercises and meditation to maintain optimum health.

- Yoga breathing exercises are both physical and spiritual in nature, intended to improve physical health, and supply the body with prana.

- The Chinese tradition of chi gong was developed as a method of moving one's vital energy (chi) around the body to ensure good health. Chi gong exercises include consciously controlled breathing.

- The meditative tradition uses conscious breathing to control moods and achieve tranquility.

- In the West, deep breathing is used by actors and singers, but anyone can learn it. You can take conscious control of your breathing for tranquility, stress management, and empowerment.

- You can learn abdominal breathing and fill your lungs completely, beginning at the diaphragm and rising to your collarbone.

*Recommended Reading*

Kaptchuk, Ted J., O.M.D. *The Web That Has No Weaver: Understanding Chinese Medicine.* Chicago: Congdon & Weed, Inc., 1983.

Hittleman, Richard. *Yoga for Health.* New York: Ballantine Books, 1983.

# *The Mind/Body*

# *Connection*

The idea that the mind plays a role in making the body ill is not new. Both Ayurveda and traditional Chinese medicine have long identified destructive emotions as the cause of many diseases. Back in the year 140 A.D. the Greek physician, Galen of Pergamum, stated that depression was a major factor in cancer. For centuries, Western medicine also believed that imbalances in the four humors of the body could be caused by severe emotions.

Not surprisingly, recent medical research has begun to uncover a great deal of scientific truth behind the mind/body connection. One aspect of this is the research done on stress and its link to serious illnesses. It is now becoming highly accepted that stress—especially how we react to it—plays a tremendous role as a causative, or contributing factor to many serious diseases.

Another aspect of the mind/body connection grows out of the new science known as *psychoneuroimmunology*, which combines the fields of psychology, neurology, and immunology. This field is discovering that emotions highly influence the chemical messengers, called *neuropeptides*, that are manufactured in our brain cells and ultimately control the immune system, and our ability to resist and fight disease.

In Part 2, we will look at the mind/body connection. We will learn about the effects of stress on the mind and body, and how to reduce or moderate reactions to stress. One of the pioneers and present day leaders in mind/body research, Dr. Carl Simonton, found that providing positive counseling to cancer patients doubles their survival rate. The work of Simonton, who developed a powerful visualization technique that has helped many cancer patients to become well, will introduce us to the exciting field of psychoneuroimmunology. Finally, we will explore nutrition for the brain; what we can do to help our central computer run at optimum efficiency, delay and prevent Alzheimer's disease, and eradicate age-associated memory impairment. In all of these responses to specific illnesses you will see considerable cross-pollination between Western and alternative medical practice.

# *Stress*

*M*aintaining vitality in the body is an important first step toward the preservation of health, and managing stress is just as important. It is estimated that 90 percent of all disease is caused or made worse by stress. While the natural healers throughout the centuries did not use the word stress, they knew extreme conditions and emotions taxed the mind and body and opened the door to disease. They observed there was a connection between severe pressure—coming from external or internal sources—and illness.

As a result, most alternative traditions have placed a high value on living a harmonized, well-balanced life that avoids stress. They also developed remedies to counter life's stressors. In this chapter, you will learn about stress and a variety of the best remedies.

Before exploring the alternative traditions, it is useful to begin with a clear understanding of the link between stress, the mind, the body, and disease.

## *Stress—a Universal Problem*

Stress is a heightened physical or mental state produced in an organism by a change in its internal or external environment.

*IN THIS CHAPTER:*

- *Stress is an unavoidable condition of life*

- *The body's response to stress*

- *Ayurvedic approaches to reducing stress*

- *Traditional Chinese medicine approaches to stress*

- *The six syllable secret in traditional Chinese medicine*

- *Alternative solutions for stress reduction*

- *Stretching techniques, progressive relaxation, and nutrition*

- *Meditation, visualization, and imagery*

Stress is even a problem for simple organisms such as yeast. Yeast responds to the stress of an increase in temperature by producing protective proteins. In humans, some of the milder stresses, such as dancing, exercise, sexual intercourse, and mental competition are regarded as beneficial.

Most of us think of stress in terms of our modern lifestyle: too many appointments, too much debt, conflicts at work, family problems. However, stress is a natural condition of the human species. Stress has been around since time immemorial, although only recently has it been truly understood from a scientific point of view.

Research conducted by Dr. Hans Selye, Robert S. Eliot, M.D., and others, has brought a new perspective to the scientific understanding of stress. Previously, stress was perceived as a result of the negative events of life. Research now shows that stress is a natural and inherent reaction of the body to *any* event or challenge that occurs. This knowledge has focused attention on a central element of stress: it is a *nonspecific* response of the body to any demand made upon it. Observations by stress researchers have led to the following conclusions:

> "Repeated incidences of stress can interfere with digestion, alter brain chemistry, increase heart rate and blood pressure, and affect metabolic and immune functioning."
>
> —Konrad Kail, N.D., past president of the American Assn. of Naturopathic Physicians

- *Stress is unavoidable.* The sheer fact of existing means the body will invariably undergo some type of stress from the simple daily events of our lives. Biologically speaking, stress includes anything and everything that makes the body react—*regardless of whether it is pleasant or unpleasant, positive or negative.* Stress can come from the environment (such as temperature), from physical or mental exertion, or from an emotion. This means your mind and/or your body can experience stress to some degree just as much from stepping out on a cold winter's day as from losing your job, or having a car accident.

- *The body is constantly adjusting* to the stressors around us to maintain its balance, or normal state of functioning. Fortunately, we are able to easily adjust to most stressors like temperature change and minor disappointments.

However, some stressors are so intense and long-lasting, they cause our mind/body to go into its adaptive mode for longer periods of time. These stressors bring about those reactions we generally call stress, but they should be more accurately dubbed distress.

• *People vary in how they react to stressors.* Some handle them very well, others do not. Researchers attributed the differences in reaction to stress to genetic heritage and environmental factors such as diet and drug usage, among others. As Dr. Selye observed, "The same stress which makes one person sick can be an invigorating experience for another."

*The Mind/Body Stress Link*

Some of the most important research in the field of stress involves what has been called the stress response. Scientists observed the body goes through three phases of response to stress:

• *Phase 1—Alarm.* The body prepares for the fight or flight response by releasing a variety of hormones that contract the muscle tissues, increase the heart rate and blood flow, and release glucose into the blood stream. The primary hormone released during this time is adrenaline, which creates the rush we feel when we are frightened, threatened, or anxious. What is important to note here is the mind is integrally involved in this phase. It must first perceive the threat for the brain to issue the orders to release the adrenaline hormones. In fact, research shows the threat does not need to be real. Even an imagined threat causes the brain to release the signal telling the adrenal glands to pump adrenaline into the blood-stream.

• *Phase 2—Resistance.* The body continues to enhance its ability to fight through the production of other hormones that stimulate additional reactions in the muscles, heart and breathing rates, blood sugar levels, and various brain centers.

*"Chi gong is the science of working with the body's energy field."*

—*Dr. Yang Jwing-ming, in* The Root of Chinese Chi Kung

• *Phase 3—Exhaustion.* The body begins to shut down to save itself from destruction from a stressor that has lasted a long time or been intense. In this phase, the body ceases producing the corticosteroids and adrenaline hormones that invigorated it during the first two phases. By this time, a certain amount of damage has been done to the body, such as depleting the cells of potassium and inhibiting the immune system from functioning properly.

---

**STRESS AND HYPERTENSION**

*One of the most frequent results of stress is hypertension, or high blood pressure. Hypertension is a serious health problem, with some 23 to 44 million Americans afflicted with it. Hypertension is dangerous because it increases the rate of development of atherosclerosis, or hardening of the arteries, which can lead to stroke and many other complications such as an enlarged heart or a diseased and shrunken kidney. These other complications occur because when the arteries are blocked, the heart pumps harder to push blood through the circulatory system, and this forces the kidneys to work harder to clean the blood. Meanwhile, the inconsistent blood flow taxes all the organs. The brain also suffers from a reduced oxygen supply, which increases the chances of a brain hemorrhage.*

*In short, the body is an astonishingly interconnected machine that can break down anywhere and at any time if subjected to too much stress.*

---

We now have an understanding of how stress, the mind, and the body are connected. On one hand, there is a clear biological link in the fact that stress causes the brain to release hormonal chemicals throughout the body that allow it to defend itself by fighting or fleeing. On the other hand, there is a significant psychological component in the fact that the stress reaction is triggered by any event the mind perceives as threatening or challenging. An event does not need to be real. As long as the mind thinks something is challenging it, it can cause the body to initiate the stress response.

Understanding that stressors can be of any quality—good or bad, positive or negative—leads to the conclusion that the mind plays a pivotal role in the stress response. As many scientists now recognize, it doesn't matter whether an event is truly stressful or not; there is no such thing as an objective rating of stress. What counts is how you perceive a stressor. If you think you will do poorly on a test or your upcoming wedding ceremony will be chaos, you can just as easily initiate the stress response as if you were about to mugged. Each person may perceive the same stressor differently, and so react differently. While one individual might handle a job interview with ease, showing no signs of nervousness or anxiety, another person might react to the same job interview with physical or psychological symptoms of stress.

### Stress and Illness

Conventional Western medicine now fully recognizes the link between stress and illness. According to studies at the National Institutes of Health, approximately 90 percent of all illnesses, both mental and physical, are caused by, or aggravated by, stress.

### Stress and Life Change

Research has shown that major life changes are often correlated with stress and resulting illness. In one study at the University of Washington Medical School, Dr. Thomas H. Holmes and Dr. Richard H. Rahe showed that major life events are often followed by illness. For example, ten times more widows and widowers die during the first year after the death of their spouse than all others in their age group.

## What Alternative Medicine Can Offer for Stress

Stress, the problems it causes and how to reduce the risks should be at the top of everyone's health list. In conventional medicine, stress is often treated with drugs, making prescription tranquilizers among the most widely used pharmaceuticals in today's society. However, alternative medicine has long offered other remedies, ranging from relaxation techniques, breathing exercises, meditation, massage, guided imagery, and visualization. Here are some specific alternative strategies for managing the stress in your life.

### The Ayurvedic Approach to Reducing Stress

Ayurveda teaches that the primary cause of stress is going against nature, as if you were attempting to swim upstream against a

---

**STRESS IS NOW HIGHLY CORRELATED WITH THE FOLLOWING DISEASES:**

Angina

Asthma

Autoimmune disease

Cancer

Cardiovascular disease

Common cold

Diabetes
(adult onset—Type II)

Depression

Headaches

Hypertension
(high blood pressure)

Immune suppression

Irritable bowel syndrome

Menstrual irregularities

Premenstrual tension syndrome

Rheumatoid arthritis

Ulcerative colitis

THE STRESS OF ADJUSTING TO CHANGE ON A
SCALE OF 1 TO 100

*"Psychological and spiritual development are capable of reversing the disease process."*
—*Dr. Bernie Siegel*

| Events & Impact | | | |
|---|---|---|---|
| Death of a spouse | 100 | Change in workload | 29 |
| Divorce | 73 | Child leaving home | 29 |
| Marital separation | 65 | Trouble with in-laws | 29 |
| Jail term | 63 | Personal success | 28 |
| Death of a family member | 63 | Spouse begins or stops work | 26 |
| Personal injury or illness | 53 | Begin or end school | 26 |
| Marriage | 50 | Change in living conditions | 25 |
| Fired at work | 47 | Trouble with boss | 23 |
| Marital reconciliation | 45 | Change in work conditions | 20 |
| Retirement | 45 | Change in residence | 20 |
| Illness in family | 44 | Change in schools | 20 |
| Pregnancy | 40 | Change in recreation | 19 |
| Sexual difficulties | 39 | Change in church activities | 19 |
| New family member | 39 | Change in social activities | 18 |
| Business readjustment | 39 | Change in sleeping habits | 16 |
| Change in financial state | 38 | Change in eating habits | 15 |
| Death of close friend | 37 | Vacation | 13 |
| Job change | 36 | Christmas | 12 |
| Foreclosure on loan | 30 | Minor violations of the law | 11 |

powerful current. Ayurvedic physicians advise that the best preventive medicine to reduce stress is to align yourself with nature's flow—that is, live in accord with natural patterns and natural law.

- Follow a daily routine that puts you in tune with the rhythms of the world. Get up early and go to bed between 9:30 and 10:30 p.m. so you can be on the same rhythm as the sun.

- Eat your largest meal at noon, when your digestive fire is the strongest.

- Get the right kind of exercise. Not only is exercise good for your heart, cardiovascular system, muscles and bones, but it is a powerful way to reduce and prevent stress. Ayurveda teaches there are different body types, and can provide specific exercise advice for each type or combination of body types.

- Avoid overfatigue. Fatigue is a form of stress. Over time, fatigue depresses the immune system, wears out the body, and produces the same harmful effects of stress.

- Avoid sensory overload. Intense sensory inputs through any of the five senses place a heavy demand on the brain and nervous system. In general, one practical way to avoid overload is to cut down on watching television and movies. They are both based on a rapid flickering of the screen, which the eye and brain accept as smooth motion due to the persistence of vision. Nevertheless, your brain is aware of being hit with 24 frames per second of film and 30 screens per second of television. Action films, TV commercials, and music videos use rapid, strobelike cuts to get your attention, along with constant and intense sound. All of these lead to a buildup of stress.

- Listen instead to relaxing music. Classical Indian music can be very soothing. There are now recordings made specifically for tranquility and meditation. Some of these incorporate the sounds of nature, the sea, the wind, and wildlife.

- Take supplements to prevent the formation of free radicals, molecules that cause extensive damage to cells and tissues.

*"Stress zaps the brain."*

—*Dharma Singh Khalsa, M.D.*

Free radicals are known to be caused by pollution, improper diet, and stress. The Ayurvedic herbal formula known as Maharishi Amrit Kalash has been found effective in reducing free radicals. Some supplements such as vitamins C and E are critical in scavenging free radicals.

---

**MANAGING DIABETES WITH YOGA**

*Type II diabetics often experience much more severe symptoms of their illness when they are under duress. As a result, some diabetes counselors now recommend the practice of yoga as an antidote to stress for diabetics. As Jon Orr, Ellen D. Davis, and Jon Seskevich, wrote in a 1995 column in Diabetes in the News: "Yoga [makes] you feel more relaxed and rejuvenated, and the tension of day-to-day life slips away. As you become less stressed, your blood glucose levels may drop. When yoga is done on a regular basis, you become better able to manage stress, which, in turn, helps you keep your blood glucose in good control."*

---

- Make time for fun and humor. Spend time each day doing something that makes you laugh, or play with your children. Taking life too seriously aggravates the stress building up in your system. Amusement and humor are great ways to diffuse stress.

### The Yoga Approach to Reducing Stress

Yoga means union. It is a holistic approach to health that focuses on one's physical, emotional, mental, and spiritual well-being. Yoga uses the body's musculature, posture, breathing, and consciousness to gain control over the mind and body. Hatha yoga, sometimes called health yoga, is widely taught and practiced in North America and Europe. It consists of breathing techniques, exercises and postures, and relaxation and meditation.

Although yoga is often considered a religious, almost mystical practice, it is gaining ground in the U. S. and in Europe as part of a healthy lifestyle for many average people seeking to relieve stress and improve physical fitness. Yoga is also gaining the respect of medical professionals in the prevention and treatment of both physical and emotional health problems.

### Traditional Chinese Medicine Approaches to Stress

Traditional Chinese medicine sees negative emotions as powerful causes of disease. The two-thousand-year-old *Internal Medicine*

*Classic* states, "If one maintains an undisturbed spirit within, no disease will occur."

"Unfortunately," says Chinese medical writer Daniel Reid, "the tendency of modern Western medicine is to treat stress with tranquilizers, which temporarily relieve the overt symptoms, but compound the physiological damage. Stress causes the adrenals to secrete adrenaline and cortisone, the latter being a particularly powerful immunosuppressant, especially in the thymus, lymph nodes, and spleen. Cortisone also impairs production of interferon, one of the body's most potent immune agents."

The primary technique by which Chinese medicine counteracts stress is through the system of physical movements known as chi gong in which conscious breathing and specific exercises regenerate vital energy, and rejuvenate the body by establishing a connection between the nervous and endocrine systems. In ancient Chinese medicine, it was believed the movements of chi gong stimulated the nerves and organs in the body, which then helped the vital energy chi to continue flowing. Modern Chinese medicine takes a similar, but more updated view, in believing that chi gong movements stimulate the central nervous system whose nerve endings extend throughout the body, many of which terminate in glands that regulate the immune system. In this way, chi gong causes a constant biofeedback loop to occur between the neurochemicals released by the nervous system and the hormones released by the immune system. Rather than having the nervous system create fight or flight hormones that cause stress, chi gong helps the nervous system produce calming, soothing neurochemicals that in turn stimulate the secretion of calming, soothing hormones. In a feedback loop, these hormones then sustain the activity of the neurochemicals, and the cycle continues.

*"By learning how to control our mind, subtle hormonal changes emerge that then control our biochemical reality."*
—*Dr. Michael Weiner,*
Maximum Immunity

## Western Approaches to Stress Reduction

Conventional Western medicine has begun to apply stress reduction techniques to patients with stress-related illnesses, such as heart disease, cancer, diabetes, and hypertension. The techniques come largely from alternative medicine, and include meditation, breathing exercises, massage, yoga, Ayurveda, and traditional Chinese medicine. Measurable changes in the physiology and health of these patients has been studied and recorded by Herbert Benson, M.D. at the Harvard Medical School and Bernie Siegel, M.D. at Yale University. Here are some answers to stress that are now meeting with success in Western medicine.

*Stretching Exercises*

One objective of stress management is to gain control over the body and the mind to avoid automatically falling into the stress response whenever you think you are being challenged or threatened. For most people, gaining control over the body is usually easier than gaining control over the mind, so stretching exercises are an excellent way to learn to take charge of your body. Stretching relieves the tension in the muscles that results from the buildup of toxins in the body. After stretching, you also feel more relaxed and in tune with yourself. You can feel your muscles and tissues, which relax from the application of the tension on them.

Many people approach stretching the wrong way, thinking that stretching is a warm up for another type of exercise. However, it is the other way around. Stretching should always be done after warming up for five to ten minutes with an aerobic workout until

---

### THE SIX SYLLABLE SECRET

*One form of ancient Chinese chi gong healing exercises is called the Six Syllable Secret, which uses the combined techniques of visualization, deep-breathing, and mind/body exercise postures to stimulate internal organs. As early as the fifth century A.D., the physician Tao-Hung-jing described this therapy in a book entitled* The Maintenance and Extension of Life.

*"One should take air in through the nose and let it out slowly through the mouth...There is one way for drawing breath in and six ways of expelling breath out. The six ways of expelling breath out are represented by the syllables chway, hsu, her, hoo, sss, shee. The six ways of exhalation can cure illness: to expel heat, use chway; to expel cold, use hoo; to relieve tension, use shee; to release anger, use her; to dispel malaise, use hsu; and to regain equilibrium, use sss."*

*The therapy is done along with easy standing postures and arm movements. Daniel Reid describes the activities of the Six Syllable Secret as follows: "The breath mobilizes energy; the lips, tongue, and throat establish the required frequency; and the movements of the limbs stimulate the associated energy channels, At the same time visualization directs the stream of energy into and out of the target organ."*

you feel warm. Stretching exercises should be done with warm muscles.

There are many ways to stretch: sitting, standing, or leaning against a wall. The first and foremost guideline is that you need to stretch your whole body to make the exercise worthwhile to you. Spend twenty minutes once a day, or at least every two or three days, to stretch your head, neck, shoulders, back, arms, and legs. Dr. Dean Ornish gives the following tips on stretching:

- The best way to stretch is without bouncing.

- Take it easy. Each movement should be slow, fluid, and controlled, as in ballet rather than calisthenics.

- Inhale as you stretch backward; exhale when you bend forward. Breathe slowly and deeply, always through your nose. Continue breathing during the stretch.

- Wait a few hours after eating before stretching.

- Remember, the process is important, not just the goal. Approach the stretches as if you were making music or dancing. What is important is to enjoy the process of stretching.

With practice, you will see that stretching can become one of the most effective components of a simple stress management program. The principles of self awareness, control over the body, and flexibility learned in stretching can later be extended to include the thoughts and emotions in a meditation program. In this sense, simple stretching with awareness is the beginning of meditation.

### Progressive Relaxation

The technique of progressive deep relaxation allows muscles to relax by first contracting them vigorously. After relaxing the mind, and a series of muscle groups, a participant in the exercise often feels a sense of well-being and ease. Others report feelings of contentment and security. The technique can be done alone or with one or more friends.

This technique was devised by Dr. E. Jacobson, a physiologist and physician, on the idea that every action has an equal and opposite reaction. Dr. Jacobson believed that tension, anxiety, stress, and related psychological problems were caused by, or made worse by, muscle contraction. He proposed the theory that muscle relaxation would have the opposite effect, relieving anxiety and mental tension. The exercise consists of lying on your back and progressively contracting and then relaxing muscle groups, starting at your feet and working up to your head. Here are some step-by-step directions on how to do the exercise. Feel free to adapt them to ways that will work for you.

**EXERCISE** *Progressive Deep Relaxation*

1. Find a quiet room. Start by lying on your back on a comfortable mat or carpet. Close your eyes. Relax your mind and your body. Focus on your breathing. You have control over your breathing. Make it deep and slow, breathing through your nose, as you would if you were beginning meditation.

2. Now focus on one part of your body, your left leg. Rock it gently. Take a deep breath, hold the breath, and raise your left leg about an inch off the floor. Squeeze and contract all the muscles in the leg and point the toe. Hold for three seconds, then relax your muscles, releasing the leg and letting it drop to the floor. As you relax your muscles, breathe out through your mouth. Breathe slowly and deeply once more. Rock your left leg gently and let it settle comfortably on the floor.

3. Focus on your right leg and repeat the exercise above with your right leg.

4. Focus your thoughts on the muscles of your pelvic region and buttocks. Breathe deeply through your nose and contract those muscles, doing a pelvic lift off the floor. Hold for three seconds, and relax, breathing out through your

mouth as you drop back to the floor. Breathe slowly and deeply.

5. Focus your thoughts on the muscles of your abdominal area. Breathe deeply through your nose. Squeeze your abdominal muscles for three to five seconds. Breathe out through your mouth as you relax. Breathe slowly and deeply after relaxing in each exercise.

6. Focus on your chest. Breathe in through your nose, expanding your chest as far as you can. Hold the breath for three to five seconds, and squeeze your chest muscles. Breathe out through your mouth as you relax.

7. Focus on your hands. Spread the fingers wide, then clench into squeezed fists. Repeat. Breathe in and contract all of the muscles in your arms as you clench fists. Raise your arms and shoulders off the floor. Relax, release your muscles, and breathe out. Relax with your palms upward and open.

8. Focus on your head and neck. Rotate your head from left to right to ease the neck. With your head centered, breathe in deeply. Hold the breath for three to five seconds while you raise your head slightly off the floor. Contract the neck muscles. Relax and breathe out.

9. Focus on your face. Relax your jaw muscles. Make a facial expression that stretches your face. Keep your eyes closed while doing this. Make an expression that squeezes your lips, nose, and eyebrows toward each other. Stretch your face. Squeeze your face. Move your face muscles from left to right and back. Relax and breathe calmly. Enjoy the tension leaving your face as if a warm scented towel was lovingly placed there by kind hands. Rotate your head from left to right to ease the neck and return to center.

10. Enjoy the relaxation in your muscles throughout your whole body. With your eyes still closed, focus your awareness on

your mind, as you would in a meditation. Allow your mental tension to release. Smile, and enjoy the relaxation of your mind. Feel the inflow of new energy as you breathe. Meditate or relax as long as you wish. Stretch and get up slowly.

## Nutrition

Dean Ornish, M.D., recommends that you try a stress-reducing diet which includes mostly fruits, vegetables, whole grains, and nonfat yogurt. This diet also benefits the heart and blood vessels because it is high in unrefined complex carbohydrates, low in cholesterol, and low in fat. Caffeine, sugar, alcohol, and processed foods should be avoided in this diet.

## Meditation

Meditation is an excellent way to regain and maintain good health without drugs. Medical studies have shown the physiological changes that take place during meditation can be measured as reductions in metabolic rate and oxygen consumption, some of them quite dramatic. These reductions slow the body down and bring it into a relaxed state that removes the products of stress.

Meditation techniques have been taught for millennia, but they all come down to four simple steps:

| EXERCISE | *Basic Meditation* |
|---|---|

1. Find a quiet place to meditate.

2. Select a simple sound or word to focus your thoughts upon. The idea of a mantra refers not to a magic word, but to a syllable that helps to clear the mind. When distracting thoughts disturb your meditation, you can return to the sound or syllable to focus your thoughts. Some people simply say the word *one.*

3. Develop a passive and receptive attitude that allows distracting thoughts or feelings to pass on by while you are centered in a place of peace.

4. A comfortable and relaxed posture. Most Westerners feel comfortable sitting on a straight chair, perhaps with a pad and a pillow to support the back. The back is straight, the head slightly raised, the hands comfortably placed in the lap, breathing is regular. If you are comfortable in other postures, please use them. Lying down is perhaps too relaxing, and may lead to sleep, a close parallel to the altered state of consciousness. The conscious breathing techniques presented in Part 1 of this book are also useful in the practice of meditation.

The ability to relax the body and the mind to such a degree that an altered state of consciousness can be achieved is a prize sought by those who practice meditation regularly.

### Visualization and Imagery

The techniques of visualization and imagery have been shown to work well when applied to stress and to healing from disease. Sometimes called applied meditation, visualization is frequently used to focus on a mental image of the desired state of health. Visualization has been a powerful tool in the alternative medicine armamentarium, proven in the pioneering work of O. Carl Simonton, M.D., his associates and patients, and many other researchers. There is now a large body of scientific evidence to support it as well. The next chapter will explain in greater detail the practice of visualization and imagery.

## Chapter Recap

- Stress is the body's reaction to any challenge or threat. When the mind perceives stress, it causes the body to go into a fight or flight mode, releasing hormones and chemicals that prepare the body to defend itself.

- Stress can be real or perceived. All that matters is that the mind believes an event is imminently challenging or threatening, and if so, it will initiate the stress response.

- Stress is a causal or contributory factor in approximately 90 percent of all illnesses, both mental and physical.

- Stress resulting from adjusting to change to major life events is often followed by illness.

- Ayurvedic remedies for stress are focused around getting in synch with the natural rhythms of life, avoiding sensory overload and fatigue, and finding time for enjoyment and humor.

- Traditional Chinese medicine sees negative emotions as powerful causes of disease. One of the major methods it recommends to relieve stress are chi gong exercises.

- Western medical recommendations to manage stress include stretching, deep-breathing techniques, nutrition, meditation, visualization, and imagery.

*Recommended Reading*

Anselmo, Peter and James S. Brooks, M.D. *Ayurvedic Secrets to Longevity & Total Health.* Englewood Cliffs, New Jersey: Prentice Hall, 1996.

Ornish, Dean M.D. *Stress, Diet & Your Heart.* New York: Holt, Rinehart and Winston, 1982.

Davitch, Victor. *The Best Guide to Meditation.* Los Angeles: Renaissance Books, 1998.

# The Mind, the Immune System, and Healing

*I*n the previous chapter, you saw how the mind plays an integral role in the link between stress and illness. But that is not the full story. Recent research reveals that the mind also plays a significant role in the operation of the entire immune system and the body's healing response. More and more studies indicate that the two work together closely, with the mind able to greatly influence how well the body succeeds in resisting disease—and even healing itself.

These studies validate many of the holistic precepts of alternative medicine. In fact, medical scientists from a variety of fields have merged to develop the field of *psychoneuroimmunology*, the new branch of science that studies the relationship between our emotions and our nervous and immune systems.

This chapter explores these psychoneuroimmunological links and presents techniques you can use to increase your resistance to disease and to heal yourself more fully and quickly.

## The Science Behind Psychoneuroimmunology

In the last two decades, medical researchers have been able to study the brain with increasing sophistication. One of their most

*IN THIS CHAPTER:*

- *The mind/body connection*
- *Endorphins in the brain affect the entire body*
- *Conscious healing through imagery*
- *The pioneering work of Dr. Carl Simonton*
- *The path of cancer and reversing the path*
- *Visualization techniques*

*145*

*"A merry heart doeth
good like a medicine,
but a bitter spirit rots
the bones."*
—*King Solomon, Proverbs*

significant findings was the existence of chemical messengers, called neuropeptides, that are produced in the brain depending on one's emotional state. These neuropeptides travel throughout the body and appear to affect a variety of chemical processes in all body systems, including the immune system. However, the kicker is some neuropeptides are manufactured in the brain only when certain emotional states of mind exist. As noted brain researcher Dr. Candace Pert of Rutgers University says, "It took us fifteen years of research before we dared to make the connection, but we know that these neuropeptides are released during different emotional states."

Some of the most interesting of these neuropeptides to be discovered are *endorphins,* which is actually short for endogenous morphines. It seems that the brain produces endorphins when there are feelings of pleasure and well-being in the mind. In fact, once the endorphins start, a positive feedback cycle occurs, because the endorphins foster the person's sense of pleasure and well-being, causing more endorphins to be released, and so on. In other words, happiness feeds upon itself.

Furthermore, the most recent studies indicate these endorphins and other neuropeptides eventually influence our immune system and ability to heal. Some studies show a correlation between the presence of neuropeptides and the ability to control blood pressure, or to heal broken bones. On the other hand, the absence of these neuropeptides, which appears to be caused by depression and negative emotions, has been shown to lead to illness.

This link between happiness and health, and sadness and ill health, actually seems quite logical and intuitive. As many alternative traditions have long held, some emotions seem to be both literally and metaphorically destructive to the body, while others seem to rejuvenate our vitality and enhance our resistance to disease. Most of us know this to be true, having had experiences in which we felt depressed or negative and then became sick. It may sound simple, but it is clearly a reflection of the body's wisdom.

## Conscious Healing through Imagery

One of the leading pioneers in the field of psychoneuroimmunology is Dr. O. Carl Simonton, M.D., a radiation oncologist who has been working with cancer patients for many years. Simonton's journey into the mind/body connection began in 1971, when he met a sixty-one-year-old patient with throat cancer. The disease was advanced, the patient could hardly swallow, and weighed only ninety-eight pounds. He was given only a 5 percent chance of surviving five years after treatment. He was already so weak that it appeared he would not respond well to radiation, so Dr. Simonton suggested the patient use visualization as well as radiation, to enhance the treatment.

The patient was given instructions on how to visualize his cancer in as vivid terms as possible. He could then use visualization, in his own way, to envision his immune system sending vast numbers of white blood cells

> **THE AMAZING IMMUNE SYSTEM**
>
> *The body's natural defense, the immune system, is one of the most important factors in whether you will be sick or well. For example, even when exposed to known carcinogens, most people remain healthy. Fortunately, exposure does not mean you will become ill. The immune system keeps people well and trouble free for years at a time.*
>
> *The immune system uses different kinds of cells to attack and destroy foreign substances in the body. An example of its action can be seen whenever pus gathers at the site of an infection. What we call pus is a mass of white blood cells that the body sends to the site to isolate and destroy the infecting microbes.*
>
> *Oncologists now believe the development of a cancer in the body requires the presence of abnormal cells, along with a suppression of the body's defense system. Theoretically, everyone at one time or another produces some abnormal cells in their body. Generally, the immune system is on the lookout for such abnormal cells and seeks them out and destroys them. This is known as the Surveillance Theory. For a cancer to take hold in the body the immune system must be, in some way, suppressed. In other words, something is happening in the people who contract cancer to allow them to become susceptible to the disease. The search for the happening event that allows susceptibility leads to the emotional and mental factors of disease or wellness. Stress is one probable cause, as are various mental and emotional problems.*

to attack and defeat the cancer cells. The patient chose to envision his white blood cells as a blizzard of white flakes, surrounding and covering the cancer tumor like snow covering a black rock. He was sent home, with instructions from Dr. Simonton to repeat the visualization at intervals on a daily basis. In a few weeks the tumor was smaller. The patient's response to radiation was nearly free of side effects. After two months, the tumor was gone. The patient went on to use visualization to solve a different problem, arthritis in his legs, and then remained free of cancer and arthritis for a follow up period of more than six years.

In 1972 Dr. Simonton received what he calls, "The gift of the world's literature." It consisted of two hundred articles on mind/body medicine. As he read through the articles he found that science and history supported the validity of this therapeutic approach. Back in the year 140 A.D. the physician Galen had already stated that depression was a major factor in cancer. Modern scientific research was rediscovering this was true. By 1981 Dr. Simonton published his first study on the effect of counseling on cancer. "Counseling," he says, "doubles the survival rate [of cancer] without side effects."

> **A SURGEON SPEAKS**
>
> *"Sir William Osler, the brilliant Canadian physician and medical historian, said that the outcome of tuberculosis had more to do with what went on in the patient's mind than what went on in his lungs. He was echoing Hippocrates, who said he would rather know what sort of person has a disease than what sort of disease a person has.*
>
> *"I personally feel that we do have biological 'live' and 'die' mechanisms within us. Other doctors' scientific research and my own day-to-day clinical experience have convinced me that the state of mind changes the state of the body by working through the central nervous system, the endocrine system, and the immune system. Peace of mind sends the body a 'live' message, while depression, fear, and unresolved conflict give it a 'die' message. Thus all healing is scientific, even if science can't yet explain exactly how the unexpected 'miracles' occur."*
>
> —Bernie S. Siegel, M.D.

### Hope, Faith, and Trust

One of the comments that people most often make about mind/body medicine is, "It's just too simple." To Dr. Simonton, these ideas are not simple, but very complex. "Mind/body medicine is as complex as the trillions of cells in a single human being. It's as intricate as we are as human beings." He goes on to say that, "Hope, faith, and trust drive the body systems to health."

### Visualization

Dr. Simonton's anticancer program is based on the premise that you can learn to control how your mind views your disease. In doing this you learn to activate your natural healing powers to fight off the cancer. Simonton's program focuses on *visualization* —a process of deep, controlled thinking using mental imagery and relaxation. The goal of your visualizations is to counteract erroneous beliefs you may have about your cancer or other illness.

Before presenting the visualization technique, it is important to understand how Simonton views the path by which cancers are believed to form in the body, as illustrated below:

Psychological stress . . . *leads to*
Depression . . . *which affects the*
Limbic System . . . *decreasing*
Hypothalamic Activity . . . *and suppressing the*
Immune System . . . *which impacts the*
Pituitary Gland and Hormonal System . . . *leading to an*
Increase in Abnormal Cells . . . *and the growth of*
Cancerous Cells

According to Simonton, this cycle of cancer development can be reversed. The pathways by which feelings can be translated into physiological conditions conducive to cancer growth can also be used to restore health. The following shows how the mind and body can interact to create health:

Psychological Intervention . . . *leads to*
Hope and Anticipation . . . *which positively affects the*
Limbic System . . . *increasing*
Hypothalamic Activity . . . *stimulating the*
Immune System . . . *increasing*
Pituitary Activity . . . *leading to a*
Decrease in Abnormal Cells . . . *and*
Cancer Regression

As Simonton and other researchers in the field of psychoneuroimmunology have discovered, patients who participate in their own recovery often have much greater psychological strength than they had before the disease. From the process of facing a life

*"The fact that the mind rules the body is, in spite of its neglect by biology and medicine, the most fundamental fact which we know about the process of life."*
—*Franz Alexander, M.D.*

threatening illness, confronting basic life issues, and learning their power to influence their health, they emerge not just restored to health, but restored with a sense of potency and control over their lives they may never have felt before the illness.

## Psychooncology

Psychooncology deals with behavioral techniques and therapies for the control of symptoms in cancer. These behavioral techniques may include hypnosis, meditation, biofeedback, progressive relaxation, and alternative methods of therapy. Most can be referred to as self-regulating therapies. In a study reported to the annual meeting of the American Psychiatric Association in May of 1989, David Spiegel, M.D., associate professor of psychiatry and behavioral sciences at Stanford Medical School described the findings of a ten-year study with cancer patients. Eighty-six women with metastatic breast cancer had been randomized into two groups. One group was given standard medical treatment alone. The other group received standard medical treatment plus weekly group therapy sessions and lessons in self-hypnosis to help control pain. The ten-year study showed that the women in the intervention group, the group that received group therapy and self-hypnosis lessons, had twice the survival time of women in the control group.

## The Effects of Spirituality and Joy on Healing

At a seminar Dr. Simonton said, "I no longer encounter resistance to using spiritual issues in any medical meeting. All of our spiritual, physical, and religious beliefs have a profound influence on our health."

Dr. Simonton also spoke about the need for joy in life. "Do more of the things that bring you joy. Mirthful laughter improves health." He urges everyone to get more enthusiasm into our life— to meditate and to imagine healthier beliefs. "Use your intellect," he said, "it is a wonderful servant, but an undesirable master."

## A Visualization to Heal a Cold                                EXERCISE

This exercise is called "The River of Life" and is adapted from Gerald Epstein, M.D. in his book *Healing Visualizations— Creating Health through Imagery:*

"Close your eyes. Breathe out three times to relax yourself. See your eyes becoming clear and very bright. Then see them turning inward, becoming two rivers flowing down from the sinuses into the nasal cavity and throat, their currents taking away all the waste products, soreness, and stuffiness. The rivers are

> **NOTE**
>
> *Visualization techniques do not replace standard medical procedures, but are to be used with them. They help patients apply, on their own, the potentially life-saving and life-extending techniques developed by researchers in psychoneuroimmunology and psychooncology. Do not delay receiving medical attention while you follow this program, which is designed to work in support of your medical treatment, not instead of it.*

flowing through your chest and abdomen, into your legs, and coming out as black or gray strands that you see being buried deep in the earth. See your breath coming out as black air and see your waste products emerging from below. Sense the rivers pulsating rhythmically through the body and see light coming from above, filling up the sinuses, nose, and throat, all the tissues becoming pink and healthy. When you sense both the rhythmic flow and light filling these cavities, breathe out, and open your eyes."

Do this exercise every three hours for three to five minutes until your cold clears up.

## Chapter Recap

- Psychoneuroimmunology is the science that studies the links between psychology, neurology, and the immune system.

- Messengers that travel throughout the body, called neuropeptides, have been shown to affect all body systems, including the immune system.

- Counseling in the practice of healthier thinking, along with visualization and imagery, can result in enhanced physical healing.

- It has been shown that negative emotions depress the immune system, lowering the body's resistance to illness, while positive upbeat emotions, like love and laughter, strengthen and empower the immune system to keep us well.

- Spirituality and joy can also help in healing.

- An exercise in healing imagery can even help with the common cold.

*"Imagine the desired*

*outcome."*

*— O. Carl Simonton, M.D.*

### Recommended Reading

Simonton, Carl, M.D., Stephanie Matthews, and James Creighton. *Getting Well Again.* Los Angeles, J.P. Tarcher Co. 1978; New York: Bantam, 1980.

Siegel, Bernie S., M.D. *Love, Medicine & Miracles.* New York: Harper & Row Publishers, 1986.

Lerner, Michael. *Choices in Healing.* Cambridge, MA: The MIT Press, 1994.

# *Brain  Food,  Brain*

# *Chemistry*

*G*iven the critical nature of the mind/body connection to your health, you would be quite correct in thinking that taking good care of your brain can make a difference in your life. Fortunately, this is one area where leading edge Western medicine excels, because of its vast understanding of neuroscience and brain chemistry.

For instance, did you know there are actually foods that can relieve anxiety and stress and help you relax? Similarly, are you aware certain natural products and vitamin and mineral supplements can significantly help your brain by enhancing your memory and your thinking powers, while others are especially good for your nervous system?

This chapter will reveal many inside tips on taking optimal care of your brain to preserve your health and increase your mental and physical performance. Just as Chapter 5 addressed the ways your vitality can benefit from the nutritional supplements A to zinc, the suggestions below will contribute to helping you live a longer, more active life for your mind—which, holistically speaking, will enhance your entire body, mind, and emotions.

*IN THIS CHAPTER:*

• *Nutrition for your brain*

• *The soothing benefits of carbohydrates*

• *Even hot chili peppers can calm you*

• *Soothing teas*

• *Vitamins, minerals, and herbs that speak to your brain*

• *Herbs for the mind and emotions*

• *Natural tonics for mental performance*

*153*

## General Nutritional Guidelines for the Brain

According to Richard Kunin, M.D., you can foster the health of your brain for optimal mental, emotional, and physical health by following these basic guidelines in choosing your nutrition:

- Eat a diet specifically suited to your body and individual needs.

- Eat natural foods, like fresh fruits, vegetables, and whole grains. Avoid processed foods.

- Eat a selection of different foods.

- Eat foods that are as free of additives and pesticides as possible. Whenever you can, choose organic foods.

- Eat in moderation—neither too much or too little.

*"Anything that helps us to cope more effectively with life, and helps us resolve emotional distress, will help our health."*

*—UCLA researcher, Fawzy I. Fawzy*

Beyond that general advice, it is worthwhile to know certain foods can benefit your mind in very specific ways. The following explains some of the best items to eat to soothe or stimulate your mind.

### The Soothing Benefits of Carbohydrates

One food group in particular, carbohydrates (which are sugars and starches) can be therapeutic to your mind and emotions in many ways. For most people, carbohydrates act as an antidepressant, relieving anxiety and stress, and increasing concentration. They also can have a tranquilizing effect, helping people relax and go to sleep.

According to Dr. Judith Wurtman, a noted food researcher at MIT, eating carbohydrates forces the insulin level to go up in your blood, which triggers a greater ratio of the chemical tryptophan. Tryptophan then quickly goes to the brain where it produces serotonin, one of the necessary neurotransmitters in the brain that helps the brain cells communicate. It turns out that serotonin soothes the brain cells, and it is thus known as the calming chemical. The more tryptophan that is supplied to the brain, the more serotonin is produced. "As a result," says Dr. Wurtman, "you feel less stressed, less anxious, more focused, and relaxed."

Some people are born with a brain chemistry that causes them to react to sugars by becoming more focused, concentrated, and alert, rather than sleepy. These people feel restless, bored, and low in energy before satisfying their craving for carbohydrates. After eating carbohydrates, they are better able to concentrate and feel calmer. When they are given a drug that increases serotonin in the brain, their cravings for carbohydrates decrease rapidly, leading to the conclusion that they lack the brain chemical serotonin.

> ### DR. JUDITH WURTMAN's CARBOHYDRATE TIPS
>
> - *Protein and fat slow down or block the process of getting serotonin to the brain. To obtain the best calming effect, eat the carbohydrate by itself, without protein and with a minimum of fat.*
> - *Some people can feel the effect of mental relief within five minutes of eating. On average, it generally takes twenty minutes or so to digest food and have the effects reach the brain. Other people may not feel the effects for an hour. To get a fast calming effect, try herbal tea with two tablespoons of cane or beet sugar.*
> - *For help with getting to sleep, try one to one and a half ounces of a sweet or starch at bedtime. For most people, this is as effective as a sleeping pill, but without the effects of morning grogginess.*

Most people, says Dr. Wurtman, need about thirty grams of pure carbohydrate to feel more tranquil. This is about the equivalent of two ounces of candy or two and a half tablespoons of sugar in the form of sucrose, cane, or beet sugar. After just the first few bites, many people will feel the effects. However, be careful, as consuming more than the minimum thirty grams doesn't help you sleep any better or relieve your stress any faster. She also notes that the kind of sugar found in fruit does not produce the same tranquilizing effect.

### Soothing Teas

Herbal teas can also produce soothing effects. Consider the following:

- *Walnut tea*—A tea made from steeping a broken half of an English walnut in boiling water, and drinking it several times a day can help raise the levels of serotonin in the body, according to Hugh Riordan, M.D. The tea is high in serotonin, says Dr. Riordan. Raising the levels of serotonin can help reduce depressive symptoms. It is also related to sleep and sensory perception.

- *Chamomile tea*—Drink a cup at night to help with insomnia, anxiety, or stress.

- *Lemon balm tea*—Drink the fresh herb as a tea for relaxation. Herbalists say lemon balm acts as an antidepressant and restorative for the nervous system.

### Hot Chili Peppers

Believe it or not, studies have revealed a number of the benefits of chili peppers, due to their active component called *capsaicin*. Chili peppers have been shown to prevent and alleviate certain lung problems, act as an expectorant, and help dissolve clots. What is more amazing though, and contrary to what you might think, is that eating chili peppers can actually soothe and calm you. As it turns out, chili peppers induce the secretion of endorphins in the brain. According to Dr. Paul Rozin, a psychologist at the University of Pennsylvania, it happens because the burning sensation or pain on the tongue and throat excites the brain to secrete endorphins to calm it.

## Brain Supplements—Vitamins, Minerals, and Hormones

While we usually think of vitamins and minerals as all-around good medicine, some are especially important nutrients for the nervous system and mental health.

### B-Complex

Taking a B50 or B100 B-complex vitamin supplement every day can help with mood swings. The B50 provides 50 mg (milligrams) of each B vitamin, and the B100 supplies 100 mg. Take one a day, or as the label directs. B vitamins are necessary for the normal functioning of the nervous system and may be the single most important factor in the health of the nerves.

### Folic Acid

A deficiency of folic acid, also called folate (which is a B-complex vitamin) has been observed to result in sleeplessness, forgetfulness, irritability, and depression. An uncomplicated way to determine if you have a deficiency is to increase the amount of folic acid in your diet to the recommended level of 400 mcg (micrograms) per day.

### Vitamin E

Several studies have shown that vitamin E supplements can reduce the severity of PMS. Researchers found that doses from 150 IU to 600 IU were successful in reducing nervous tension, moodiness and mood swings, confusion, crying, depression, irritability, anxiety, insomnia, cravings, and memory loss. The recommended daily allowance (RDA) for vitamin E is 30 IU. However, medical experts suggest a dose for most healthy people of 400 IU per day.

### Calcium and Magnesium

Calcium can act as a sleep aid when taken at bedtime. You can buy capsules that have a ratio of twice the amount of calcium to the amount of magnesium. Magnesium is another naturally calming mineral that works with calcium in many ways. The RDA for calcium is 1,200 mg for ages 11–24, and 800 mg above age 24. Medical experts recommend 800–1,000 mg of calcium (citrate) and 350–500 mg of magnesium (citrate, gluconate, or chelate) at bedtime.

### Melatonin

Melatonin is a hormone secreted by the pineal gland, a small gland located in the brain. Early researchers thought the gland resembled a pine cone, hence they named it pineal. The pineal gland in all mammals secretes the hormone melatonin during the dark phase of the body's circadian cycle, our daily sleep/wake cycle that moves in roughly twelve hour periods. Melatonin levels peak during childhood, and decline with age. The steepest decline begins at about age fifty. By age sixty, say researchers, our pineal glands are producing half the melatonin they did when we were twenty. Not so coincidentally, as melatonin levels drop, we begin to exhibit signs of aging.

As a result of these findings, many researchers now recommend melatonin to aid in sleep and relaxation. It is available in health food stores. Some people use it as a sleeping pill. Two medical researchers who recommend melatonin, are Walter Pierpaoli, M.D., Ph.D. and William Regelson, M.D. Their book, *The Melatonin Miracle,* with co-author Carol Colman, describes melatonin as "Nature's age-reversing, disease-fighting, sex-enhancing hormone." They sum up its benefits as follows:

- Age reversing, "Melatonin can extend our lives by decades while keeping our bodies young."

- Disease fighting, "Melatonin can help prevent heart disease, cancer, and other common diseases."

- Stress relieving, "Melatonin can protect us from the destructive effects of chronic stress."

- Sleep cycle restoring, "Melatonin is a safe, nonaddictive sleeping agent that can cure disruptions in our sleep/wake cycle, such as jet lag and insomnia."

- Sex enhancing, "Moreover, melatonin promises not only to maintain and restore an interest in sex, but, our research has shown, it actually helps to rejuvenate sex organs."

The doses of melatonin taken at bedtime recommended by Drs. Pierpaoli and Regelson are adjusted by age.

MELATONIN RECOMMENDATIONS

| Age | Quantities |
| --- | --- |
| 40–44 | .5 to 1 mg |
| 45–54 | 1 to 2 mg |
| 55–64 | 2 to 2.5 mg |
| 65–74 | 2.5 to 5 mg |
| 75 plus | 3.5 to 5 mg |

A Dallas, Texas, physician, William Lee Cowden, M.D. suggests taking melatonin capsules nightly, between 10:00 p.m. and midnight, for one or two weeks to "reset the biological clock," then take them every other night for several months until your sleep habits are normalized.

There are two forms of melatonin available: synthetic forms and the so-called natural melatonin, made from the extract of animal pineal glands. Many scientists prefer and recommend synthetic melatonin as its dosage level can be more accurately controlled.

### CAUTIONS ABOUT MELATONIN

*Medical experts do not recommend melatonin supplementation for children. Melatonin is also not recommended for women during pregnancy and lactation. Increasing a mother's melatonin level increases the amount delivered to the fetus, which is not warranted. Anyone taking prescription medications should check with their physician before using melatonin. Carefully follow all directions.*

### DHEA

The letters DHEA stand for a hormone made by the adrenal glands, called dehydroepiandrosterone (pronounced dee-hi-dro-ep-E-an-dro-stehr-own). DHEA supplements are available in health food stores. Researchers claim DHEA is a means to boosting sex drive, enhancing energy, mood, and memory, and improving the immune system.

Of the more than one hundred and fifty hormones which are synthesized by our adrenal glands, the most abundant is DHEA. Once it reaches the bloodstream, DHEA travels to cells throughout the body where it is converted into male hormones called androgens, or female hormones, called estrogens, depending on certain factors. Both men and women have some of each of these two hormones, but the amounts vary depending on the age, gender, and medical condition of the person.

If the benefits of DHEA supplements are important to you, it is a subject well worth discussing with your physician. It can aggravate certain health problems in some people, such as prostate conditions in men.

## Herbs for the Mind and Emotions

Most of us are quite familiar with using herbs like basil, rosemary, and thyme in our cooking. Those of us who have a beer once in a while have no problem ingesting hops. Some of us who scent our home with lavender know what a wonderful smell it can impart. Well, if you are already doing such things with herbs, it's only a small leap to using herbs to ease your mind and emotions. The following sections reveal the beneficial brain effects of certain herbs.

### Basil (Ocimum basilicum)

Basil acts as an antidepressant and is uplifting to the spirit. You can eat the fresh leaves, or add five drops of basil essential oil to your bath water, or take up to 3 ml of a basil tincture three times a day. You can also take it as an infusion, made much like tea. Pour boiling water in a pot with a lid. Leave basil leaves to infuse ten minutes, strain into a teacup, and drink hot or cold.

### Hops (Humulus lupulus)

Hops are good for insomnia. They are a sedative and calm excitability. Add 10 grams of the herb to 500 ml of water for an infusion at night. Do not exceed the stated dose. However, don't take hops for depression.

### Lavender (Lavandula)

In addition to its beautiful flower, lavender helps you relax. It is a sedative and an analgesic. You can make an infusion, or you can take up to 4 ml of the tincture per dose. The essential oil, which is concentrated, needs to be diluted and is not for internal use. It mixes well with carrier oils, moisturizers such as aloe vera, or with chamomile cream or a little water. Use one drop of essential oil to about fifteen drops of carrier oil. Massage the diluted oil into your temples, and you will love the aroma. Avoid high doses of lavender if you are pregnant.

### Ginkgo Biloba

Many people have heard about ginkgo biloba recently, because the herb has become very popular for its ability to help you think more clearly and have an improved memory. What is the truth about this? Indeed, it turns out that ginkgo biloba does have beneficial effects on the brain.

The active ingredients in ginkgo are flavonoids, which you might recall from Chapter 5 are natural chemicals in many plants, including citrus fruits, that have aspirin like qualities of constricting the blood vessels and improving circulation. Ginkgo also contains flavonglycocides, which are part of the bioflavonoid family, but are flavonoid molecules unique to ginkgo biloba, and terpenes, particularly Ginkgolide B, another chemical found in many plants such as ginseng. One researcher discusses the value of ginkgo as helping to "scavenge free radicals and inhibit the platelet activating factor (PAF). Both free radical formation and PAF can disrupt vascular membranes, resulting in increased vascular permeability which in turn is associated with the impairment of blood flow seen with aging."

In a study of ginkgo at Whittington Hospital in London, improved brain function was found in a group of thirty-one patients over age fifty with signs of memory impairment. Half the volunteers were given 40 mg of ginkgo biloba extract (GBE) three times a day, while the other half remained on placebo. At the end of twenty-four weeks the researchers reported that: "The patients who received GBE showed significantly superior improvement compared to those given a placebo. Besides demonstrating that ginkgo extract has a beneficial effect on mild to moderate memory loss of organic origin, the study revealed that electroencephalogram (EEG) measurements in the GBE group indicated improved brain function. This supports other research that GBE increases the rate of information transmission by nerve cells."

It is the leathery, fan shaped leaves of the ginkgo biloba tree, also known as the maidenhair tree, that are used in producing the extract found in commercially prepared capsules. The graceful trees can top one hundred feet, with trunks eight feet in diameter, and can reportedly live for over a thousand years. They were widely distributed over the temperate regions during the time of the dinosaurs, and date back over two hundred million years. The ice age reduced their numbers, but they survived in China and Japan, where they have been cultivated for millennia. They are now widely planted as ornamentals in temperate climates. Extracts of ginkgo leaves are widely used in both European and Asian medicine.

Researchers generally recommend a dosage of 120 mg per day in divided doses of 40 mg three times a day. Directions for the 60 mg tablets are usually one tablet twice per day, preferably once in the morning and once in the late afternoon or early evening, with or before meals. Follow the directions on the label for the potency you select.

### St. John's Wort (Hypericum perforatum.)

Wort is an old English word for plant. The St. John's in the name may have come from the Knights of St. John, who treated pilgrims to the Holy land with external applications of the herb, which are known to reduce pain and inflammation. Some people prefer to call this useful herb by its botanical name, Hypericum.

Of interest is its reputation for enhancing mood and lifting the spirits. Taken internally, the leaves and flowers of Hypericum can lighten the mood and lift the spirits. Some call the plant a restorative nerve tonic ideal for anxiety and irritability, especially during menopause. Hypericum is also good for chronic, long-standing conditions where nervous exhaustion is a factor. An infusion, or tea, can be made by pouring boiling water over the dried leaves and flowers of the plant.

Extracts of Hypericum are licensed in Germany for the treatment of anxiety and depressive and sleep disorders. It is considered among the seven most popular preparations in Germany, and in 1993 more than 2.7 million prescriptions for Hypericum were written.

**CAUTIONS WITH ST. JOHN'S WORT**

*Even St. John's Wort extract, standardized to 0.3 percent Hypericum, can be dangerous to some. Most bottles will tell you not to use Hypericum if you are pregnant, lactating, or taking antidepressant medications. It is also known that you should limit your exposure to the sun when taking St. John's Wort as it is known to cause increased photosensitivity in fair skinned individuals. In addition, in* The Complete Medicinal Herbal, *herbalist Penelope Ody notes the herb can cause dermatitis after taking it internally, and exposing the skin to the sun.*

## Nutrition and Natural Tonics for Mental Performance

Loss of memory performance has long been associated with aging. Dharma Singh Khalsa, M.D. is a self-described baby boomer, who developed a fascination about brain longevity after many fellow boomers—people in their fifties—came to him seeking help for memory impairment. His approach integrates both conventional and alternative medicine, a combination he calls integrative medicine.

Much of what Dr. Khalsa recommends would be classified as natural tonics, substances that tonify or strengthen the function of a body system. Even if the system is already functioning at normal levels,

> **MEMORY AND AGING**
>
> *Writing about a loss of memory that one baby boomer was lamenting to him, Dr. Khalsa writes in his book,* Brain Longevity: *"I knew full well what [my patient] was talking about. I often heard similar versions of the same complaint. I even had a name for it: The Cry of the Wounded Boomer. . . . Baby boomers, who were just now hitting the memory barrier of their late forties and early fifties, were consulting me with increasing frequency. They were shocked by the sudden onset of age-associated memory impairment, and by the corresponding declines in their hormonal systems. They were suddenly losing the mental sharpness . . . and needing more and stronger coffee just to slog through the day. The boomers' loss was Starbuck's gain."*

tonics can improve that functioning. "Modern Western medicine pays little attention to improving normal function," says Dr. Khalsa. "In Eastern medicine, however, tonics play a major role. So even if you feel your cognitive function is normal, you should try some of these tonics. They may lift you to a new level."

The following sections list some of Dr. Khalsa's natural and nutritional recommendations for tonics that can provide a lifetime of peak mental performance.

### Lecithin

Many persons already ingest about 1,000 mg of lecithin daily as part of their natural diet, but this is not a high enough quantity to promote brain longevity. According to Dr. Khalsa, lecithin's active ingredient, phosphatidyl choline, is the nutritional building material for acetylcholine, the primary neurotransmitter of thought and memory. "Lecithin is nontoxic," says Dr. Khalsa, "and may be taken in very high dosages without side effects. A reasonable dosage would be about 1,500 mg daily, for a person with no significant cognitive impairment. If early-stage memory impairment is present, this dosage can be doubled or tripled."

### Phosphatidyl Serine (PS)

An extremely beneficial brain tonic, phosphatidyl serine (abbreviated as PS) is found in lecithin. It is not easily found in other common foods, but is available in capsule form in most health food stores. PS is derived from soy lecithin. According to Dr. Khalsa, "Many of my patients report to me that PS has had a dramatic, positive effect upon their cognitive function. A reasonable dosage for a brain longevity patient would be 100 to 300 mg daily, depending upon the patient's degree of cognitive decline. Anything less than 100 mg is ineffectual."

### Acetyl L-Carnitine (ALC)

A naturally occurring substance that aids cognition, ALC improves energy metabolism in the brain. It also reduces generation of free radicals in the cells. Dr. Khalsa says, "ALC also has the fascinating ability to improve communication between the two hemispheres of the brain. When this improvement to communication occurs, it spurs creativity and helps the patients achieve a more balanced cognitive ability." He cited a study where subjects were tested on their ability to travel through a maze and find the exit. After they were given ALC, the time it took them to exit the maze was reduced by 43 percent.

ALC is expensive. A bottle of one hundred capsules with 500 mg each costs about $75. "For many of my patients, I prescribe 250 mg of ALC daily," says Dr. Khalsa. He strongly recommends patients take ALC with phosphatidyl serine (PS) because the two substances potentiate each other.

### Ginseng

Dr. Khalsa endorses ginseng for its astonishing neurological effects. He too points out that the herb works on the hormonal system, stopping the overproduction of cortisol. "Cortisol is an excitatory hormone, like adrenaline, but stays in the system longer and is more disruptive," Dr. Khalsa says. "Unrelenting stress causes production of cortisol in the brain. The best way to handle cortisol is to manage your stress. The amount of cortisol that bathes the memory center of the brain over a lifetime does the damage, like that found in Alzheimer's disease." Studies show that students using ginseng have greatly improved their scores on cognitive function tests. The herb has been shown to increase mental and physical stamina and help to resist stress-related diseases.

Among the different varieties of ginseng, Dr. Khalsa recommends Siberian ginseng, in a reasonable daily dosage of 750 mg to 1,500 mg, depending upon your medical condition and the quality of ginseng.

### Green Juice Products

Green juice products include blue-green algae, barley grass, chlorella, oat grass, spirulina, and wheat grass. "These products are of particular value to brain longevity patients," says Dr. Khalsa, "because they include combinations of amino acids (or partial proteins) called peptides, which can be transformed into neuropeptides." Neuropeptides, such as beta-endorphins, are one of the primary links between mind and body. Green juice products are also rich in essential amino acids. Two of these amino acids, tryptophan and phenylalanine, are the building blocks for the important neurotransmitters serotonin and norepinephrine. As Dr. Khalsa writes, "I advise patients to take their green juice product first thing in the morning, as part of their wake up routine. Many of my patients who use a green juice product report a noticeable increase in their cognitive abilities, as well as an increase in their general levels of well-being.

"The vast majority of the above listed nutrients are appropriate for all patients, even when taken in high dosages. Further, all of these nutrients at moderate levels are absolutely vital for all people. Your brain has always needed each one of them, and always will."

DAILY DOSAGES OF NUTRITIONAL SUPPLEMENTS
FOR BRAIN LONGEVITY

| Nutrient | Quantities |
|---|---|
| Vitamin A | 10,000–25,000 IU |
| Vitamin B12 | 100–1,000 mcg |
| Vitamin B6 | 50–200 mg |
| Vitamin B1 | 50–100 mg |
| Folic Acid | 400 mcg |
| Niacin | 100–200 mg |
| Vitamin B5 | 100–200 mg |
| Vitamin C | 3,000 mg |
| Vitamin E | 400–800 mg |
| Magnesium | 200–300 mg |
| Selenium | 50–100 mcg |
| Zinc | 30–50 mg |
| Multi vitamin/mineral | 1–2 tablets (May contain all of the above) |
| Amino acids | One serving, protein powder |

## Chapter Recap

- Many foods and supplements can help the brain improve its memory, functioning, and general health.

- Carbohydrates can be therapeutic to the mind and emotions in many ways.

- For soothing teas try walnut, chamomile, and lemon balm.

- Vitamins and minerals important to the nervous system are B-complex, folic acid, vitamin E, magnesium, and calcium.

- For a sleep aid, consider melatonin. Check the recommended dosages by age, and read the cautions.

- Ginkgo biloba extract is being used for improved memory and brain function, and acts as an antioxidant.

- Herbalists say that Hypericum (St. John's wort) can lighten the mood and lift the spirits.

- Dr. Dharma Singh Khalsa recommends a variety of natural tonics to stimulate the brain and increase its performance.

*Recommended Reading*

Khalsa, Dharma, Singh, M.D. *Brain Longevity—The Breakthrough Medical Program That Improves Your Mind and Memory*. New York: Warner Books, 1997.

Murray, Frank. *Ginkgo Biloba: The Amazing 200 Million Year Old Healer*. New Canaan, CT: Keats Publishing, Inc., 1993.

Ody, Penelope. *The Complete Medicinal Herbal*. London: Dorling Kindersley, 1993.

# Prevention and

# Longevity

Why is it that some people can be exposed to germs and not get sick, or be in contact with carcinogens and not get cancer? Why do some people live healthy lives until they are in their 90s, while others succumb to debilitating illnesses that take the joy out of their lives at seventy-three? The answers to these questions lie in whether or not someone follows a lifestyle that promotes health and longevity.

Western science teaches, on one hand, that disease prevention is a function of the immune system, the complex defenses the body has to ward off illness or injury. In the following chapters, you will learn how the immune system works, how the latest discoveries of alternative medicine can help you strengthen it, and how you can develop an anticancer and antiheart disease lifestyle that will help you live longer and enjoy life more.

The traditional Chinese medical view holds that our life span should be at least one hundred years. With that goal in mind, what can alternative medicine do to keep you living longer and loving it?

# *Disease Prevention and Your Immune System*

*A*s you have seen in the previous sections, the concept of maintaining your health and preventing disease before it occurs is central to alternative healing therapies. While the older traditions may not possess the scientific understanding to pinpoint prevention as a function of the immune system, practitioners knew the body had some type of natural mechanism which, if maintained properly, would keep illness away. When illness did strike, it seemed to defend itself and attempt to throw off the disease. This is why many alternative traditions attempt to rebalance the vital energy system of the body through gentle medications, nutrition, and exercise, rather than attacking the disease itself.

In its search for a more scientific explanation of the body's disease prevention and healing mechanisms, convention Western medicine has focused on the workings of the body's immune system. Increasingly sophisticated analysis has revealed when health is threatened, the body produces a wide assortment of cells, hormones, and chemicals to seek out and destroy the foreign invaders, and still others to strengthen and repair any injury or debilitation. This is only one of the amazing facts from the leading edge of immunological research with profound implications for health and wellness.

*IN THIS CHAPTER:*

- *The immune system as your first line of defense*

- *Bacteria, viruses, and free radicals*

- *Alternative methods of protecting the immune system*

- *Sex and the immune system*

- *Naturopathic medicine and natural healing*

- *Vitamin and mineral protectors*

- *Aromatherapy and baths*

- *Western medicine and antioxidants*

- *Natural food sources of antioxidants*

## The Immune System—Your First Line of Defense

The immune system is the star performer in the lifelong quest to maintain a defense against disease. Western medicine has learned the immune system consists of such organs and glands in the body, including the tonsils and adenoids, the thymus gland, the lymph nodes throughout the body, the bone marrow, the circulating white blood cells and other cells that leave blood vessels to migrate through tissues and the lymphatic circulation, the spleen, the appendix, and patches of lymphoid tissue in the intestinal tract.

The immune system is a complex system of warriors and messengers that coordinate across and throughout every level of the body. The first line of defense begins with specialized scout cells that roam the body seeking out anything foreign or harmful, such as invading bacteria, damaged and infected cells, and tumor cells. When any threat or injury is detected, the scout cells send messengers to the endocrine system, which then goes into action by releasing other specialized cells designed to attack any source of infection or toxin.

## Anatomy of an Immune System

If you could look inside the immune system you would find at its basis, the lymphatic vessels which run throughout every organ except the brain, circulating lymph fluid and white blood cells, star players in our body's first line of defense. The lymph system runs through every organ except the brain. Situated along the vessels of the lymphatic system are specialized areas involved in creating the various cells and chemicals used in the body's defense.

### White Blood Cells

Most of the cells you will encounter in the immune system are different types of white blood cells. These include macrophages, neutrophils, and lymphocytes.

- *Lymphocytes*—The principle cells of the immune system. There are two types of lymphocytes:

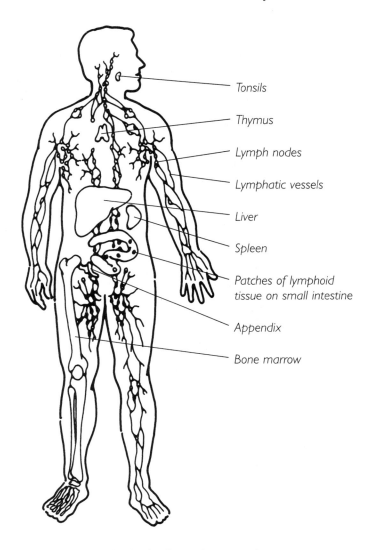

Tonsils

Thymus

Lymph nodes

Lymphatic vessels

Liver

Spleen

Patches of lymphoid tissue on small intestine

Appendix

Bone marrow

*Type T lymphocytes*—Enable the body to distinguish self from non-self, thereby targeting foreign invaders, which could be microbes, transplanted organs, or cancer cells.

*Type B lymphocytes*—Function to produce antibodies.

- *Macrophages*—Large cells that engulf and ingest microbes that have been identified as invaders by the immune system.

- *Natural killer cells*—Another kind of lymphocyte that is capable of killing cancer cells and certain microbes. They are referred to as natural because they are ready to kill invading cells as soon as they form and do not need the education and maturation process required by T and B lymphocytes.

- *Neutrophils*—Ingest antigens and other substances that are targeted for removal.

*Fighting Bacterial Infections, Viruses, and Free Radicals*
The body's enemies can be divided into several major camps, such as bacteria, viruses, and oxidized free radicals. Each type of invader differs in its methods of attacking the body, its method of reproduction, and its manner of survival against the body's attempt to rid itself of the invader.

- *Bacteria*—Disease-causing microscopic, single-cell organisms that lack a distinct nucleus, usually reproduce by cell division, and can be found in nearly all environments. About two hundred species of bacteria are known to cause disease in humans. Their strength and danger vary widely. Bacteria are responsible for the following diseases: cholera, lockjaw, gangrene, leprosy, plague, dysentery, tuberculosis, syphilis, typhoid fever, diphtheria, and many forms of pneumonia. Until the discovery of viruses, bacteria were considered the cause of all infectious diseases. Bacteria can be driven from the body by the immune system or antibiotic drugs which kill them.

- *Free Radicals*—Tiny, submicroscopic oxygen molecules with a defect of an unpaired electron that makes them unstable. Oxygen is necessary for normal functioning of the human body, but there are two kinds of oxygen molecules, stable and the unstable radicals. Without the stable oxygen molecules, life could not exist. The unstable molecules have their own uses. In proper balance, free radicals fight inflammation, kill bacteria, and tone the muscles that regulate internal organs and blood vessels. However, when there is an excess of unstable oxygen molecules in the body, it creates disaster. Free radicals have been implicated in triggering a variety of diseases including cancer, heart disease, premature aging, atherosclerosis, and cataracts.

It is not known why free radicals form, but they cause the body's oxidation process to go haywire, to inflict irreparable damage to DNA in cells. An oxygen molecule that is a free radical enters the body—from, for example, rancid oil used in cooking french fries—and takes an electron from a stable molecule. This causes the previously stable molecule to become a free radical. It, in turn, seeks out and steals an electron from yet a different stable molecule causing the third molecule to become a free radical. In the process, permanent DNA damage has been done to each molecule. (In other words, the process of stealing a molecule does not heal or repair.) The continuing process of stealing an electron initiates a chain reaction of destructiveness. Because free radicals have one or more unpaired electrons in their outer orbits, they act as magnets that must grab onto something in a vain attempt to regain their stability. Free radicals dart throughout the cells of the body like jalopies in a demolition derby, crashing into other particles and tissues, stressing the tissues and ultimately organs.

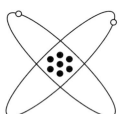

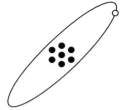

*Stable molecules have electrons that are in pairs. The electrons hold the molecules together.*

*Unstable molecules have an electron that does not have a pair. The molecule becomes reactive and unstable—a free radical.*

- *Viruses*—Submicroscopic parasites that consist of the genetic material RNA or DNA plus a protective coating of protein are viruses, another cause of infectious diseases. They reproduce only in actively metabolizing cells. Outside of a living cell, viruses exist only as inert macromolecules. The common cold is perhaps the most widespread viral disease. Other viral diseases include influenza, measles, mumps, chicken pox, shingles, fever blisters, respiratory diseases, acute diarrhea, warts, and hepatitis. Life-threatening diseases caused by a virus include rabies, hemorrhagic fevers, encephalitis, poliomyelitis, and yellow fever. Increasing evidence indicates that viruses may be the basis of some types of cancer, along with chronic and degenerative diseases such as multiple sclerosis and Creutzfeldt-Jakob disease. Viruses can be spread by airborne particles expelled when people sneeze or cough, through fecal-oral contamination, or by insects. They can remain in the body for a long time before acting. Many viruses cannot be destroyed by drugs because the drugs also kill cells in which the viruses live. One effective means of preventing viral illnesses is vaccination. Vaccines stimulate the immune system to produce antibodies which are already in the body and prepared to attack the specific RNA or DNA of a virus when it first appears. Otherwise, the only ways to eliminate viruses once they enter the body are natural remedies and time.

## The Role of Free Radicals in Disease and Aging

When the body has too many extra free radicals, these molecular outlaws can run wild, attacking healthy tissue as well as invading bacteria. The results are serious. Heart disease, atherosclerosis, cancer, cataracts, some forms of arthritis, and premature aging can all be traced back in some way to free radical activity. Some triggers of excess free radicals can be found in the environment: cigarette smoke, air pollution, pesticides, contaminants in food, radiation, even the ultraviolet light that comes from the sun. The ozone we breathe in from vehicle exhaust, for example, is a highly reactive air pollutant that has been observed to form free radicals in the lungs.

Researcher David J. Lin describes some body systems, in the following sections, which are affected by free radicals.

### Aging

The accumulation of free radical damage to the body's cells over time appears to be a key factor in aging. Moreover, says David Lin, aging itself may be the result of diminished ability to balance and control free radicals, which may increase the risk of disease. One proof of this is that antioxidant supplements have been shown to boost the function of the immune  system in the elderly.

### Atherosclerosis

Deposits of plaque on the inside of blood vessels can obstruct normal blood flow leading to coronary heart disease. Normal cholesterol, which has long been blamed for the creation of plaque in blood vessels, may not be the only culprit. Oxidized cholesterol, which has been damaged by free radicals, may play the most important role forming plaque in the arteries of the heart.

### Cataracts

Ultraviolet light radiation can enter the eye and form free radicals in the eye tissues. These free radicals may then damage proteins in the lens, causing them to cross link and precipitate out as solid, opaque masses. The fluids of the eye contain very high levels of antioxidants, nutrients that combat free radicals. Without this protection, the eyes would be even more vulnerable to free radical damage. High quality sunglasses, which can screen out radiation, should always be worn for protection. Eye protection and adequate levels of antioxidant supplements are recommended as prudent protection for the eyes.

### Joint Disease and Arthritis

The synovial fluid, the fluid providing cushioning between bones, can be invaded by free radicals, causing inflammation. When the area becomes inflamed, the body's immune cells rush to the damaged area, producing more free radicals.

## Protecting the Immune System in Alternative Medicine

Many alternative healing traditions make a high priority of protecting the body against the forces that deplete it of its ability to fight disease. While Ayurveda, Chinese medicine, and naturopathy did not possess the scientific understanding of our immune system and the glands and tissues that produce antibodies to fight disease, they did understand the important role physical vitality plays in maintaining the body's ability to fight disease and prevent disease from striking. In this sense, all their recommendations

### AYURVEDIC AND CHINESE METHODS OF RESISTING DISEASE

| *The Ayurvedic Way of Prevention* | *The Chinese Way of Prevention* |
| --- | --- |
| A balanced lifestyle, in harmony with your personal constitution; moderation in all things; staying in tune with nature. | A balanced lifestyle that avoids exhaustion, overeating, extremes of hot and cold, and destructive emotions; living in harmony with the yin and yang energies of the universe. |
| Nutrition—eat according to your dosha. Moderation, mostly a vegetarian diet, with certain other foods believed to foster immunity, such as milk, rice, honey, and ghee. | Nutrition—eat fresh foods, in moderation, mostly focusing on vegetables, rice, fish, and small amounts of meat. |
| Use rejuvenating herbs (rasayanas) and tonics that promote health and keep the digestive system in good balance, such as winter cherry, garlic root, Indian asparagus, fo-ti, and licorice. | Use tonic herbs to rejuvenate the body and revitalize the chi (vital energy); main Chinese herb was ginseng. |
| Energy work—yoga or exercise positions (asanas). | Energy work—chi gong and other movement exercises. |
| Deep breathing exercises and meditation. | Deep breathing via various exercises that focused on controlling the mind and body. |
| Sexual moderation to preserve one's prana (vital energy). | Sexual moderation to preserve your chi. |

aimed at increasing vitality are focused on strengthening and protecting the immune system.

The chart on page 178 provides a summary of the many similar views that Chinese and Ayurvedic medicine shared concerning the maintenance of vitality and the prevention of illness.

*"Only nature heals."*
—*The School of Hippocrates*

### Sex and the Immune System

Ayurvedic medicine considers the body's sexual energy to be reflective of its immune system's state of vitality. In Ayurveda, the essential energy of the body is called *ojas*. Ayurveda holds that ojas is depleted by overwork, stress, anxiety, poor diet, inadequate sleep, use of drugs, and excessive sex. When you are low on ojas, you are susceptible to disease.

To remain healthy, Ayurvedic medicine advises you to rejuvenate your ojas regularly. To further this rejuvenation, Ayurveda recommends two types of herbs that are intended to promote vitality and virility. One group of herbs, *vijakarasana*, are tonics to rejuvenate the sexual organs where the reproductive tissue is thought to be the source of all creation in the body. The second group of herbs are the *rasayanas*, which were described in the chapter on vitality. They are the Indian equivalent of Chinese ginseng, tonic herbs that were believed to promote vitality and enhance immunity throughout the body.

If you feel low in sexual energy, Ayurveda warns that your immune system may also be operating at a low level. Among the possible tonic herbs Ayurveda recommends are: tang kwei, wild yam, licorice, ginseng, saffron, cloves, and saw palmetto. One traditional concoction available from Ayurvedic herbalists, *Chayavanapransha*, is made up of thirty to fifty different herbs which are full of iron, calcium, silica, sodium, potassium, phosphates, plant sterols, and vitamin C. One of the main herbs is *amla*, the most respected of all Ayurvedic tonics, that is believed to increase ojas, rejuvenate the body, and increase the sexual drive.

## Naturopathy, Immunity, and Healing

Naturopathy focuses heavily on the body's natural ability to resist disease and heal itself.

Naturopathy dates back to Hippocrates. Like Ayurvedic medicine and traditional Chinese medicine, it is based on the belief that the body has a vital life that must remain in balance for health. Naturopathy is a holistic system, viewing the body, mind, and spirit as equal partners in determining the state of health in each person. What affects the body, also affects the mind—and vice versa.

A healthy, balanced life along with the right foods and emotional conditions fosters a healthy state that helps the body resist disease and even heal itself. Naturopathy believes that the flow of life's energies is toward preserving health and the cells of the body are primed to stay healthy and to fight illness to preserve themselves.

The founder of modern naturopathy, Benedict Lust, a German who emigrated to the United States in 1896, was dedicated to working solely with the realm of the body's own natural rhythms and powers. He formulated the first modern program for naturopathic doctors in New York in 1902. It consisted of botanical medicine, nutritional therapy, physiotherapy, psychology, homeopathy, and manual manipulation techniques such as massage. Over the next few decades, naturopathy achieved a condition of predominance in medicine, but faded between the 1940s and 1980s, only to be rediscovered again recently and undergo a resurgence.

Today, naturopathy teaches that disease is brought on by a variety of conditions endemic to modern life. One is the change of diet from unrefined fresh foods to refined and processed foods. Unresolved mental stress created by our work and social environment is another cause. Toxins resulting from environmental pollution are also seen as contributing to disease. Other hindrances to health identified by naturopathy are:

- Accumulation of toxic material within the body

- Destructive emotions

- Excessive use of tobacco, alcohol, and caffeine

*"Naturopathy is a method of curing disease by releasing inner vitality and allowing the body to heal itself."*

*—Dr. Ross Trattler*

- Improper posture and body mechanics

- Incorrect or unbalanced diets

- Inherited factors

- Mental and emotional stress

- Occupational hazards and work-related stress

- Pollution of the air, water, and soil

- Suppressive drugs

- Viral and bacterial infections

Naturopathy teaches that when one or more of these factors exist, the body is forced to act vigorously to reestablish correct equilibrium. The result is acute disease.

### The Six Principles of Healing

To counter disease, traditional naturopathy is based on six principles of healing:

- *The healing power of nature*—The body has a natural healing power, and the physician must identify the blockages preventing the body's own healing powers from working.

- *Treat the whole person*—The body is an intricate web of forces whose harmonious functions determine health. Disease is an imbalance in one part that affects the whole. Therapy must therefore aim to create the whole person by restoring the proper balance.

- *Do no harm*—The body should be protected from harmful side effects by using gentle and noninvasive therapies.

- *Identify and treat the cause*—Symptoms are not the cause of illness, but an expression of the body's attempt to heal itself. The underlying causes of disease are found in the patient's lifestyle, diet, habits, or emotional state.

- *Prevention is best cure*—The patient is shown how to take steps to prevent the onset of disease by choosing the proper lifestyle.

- *The doctor is a teacher*—The physician teaches the patient self-responsibility.

### The Tools of Naturopathy

The medical tools of naturopathy depend upon the choices of the individual naturopath, and may include the following:

- *Herbal medicine*—The use of herbal substances, like Chinese and Ayurvedic medicine, are found to have the power to stimulate the body's own resources to combat disease.

- *Homeopathy*—The use of homeopathic remedies based on the principle of "like cures like." This involves using natural herbal potions that create a certain symptom to cure the same symptom in an ill person. Because they are natural, extremely minute doses are used.

- *Hydrotherapy*—The use of hot and cold water treatments to stimulate the circulatory and immune system to action.

- *Nutritional therapy and fasting*—The use of nutrition and fasting to stimulate the body's natural disease resistance powers, and maintain the immune system in optimal condition.

- *Spinal manipulation*—The use of chiropractic and massage therapies to stimulate the nerves and loosen toxins from bodily tissues, based on the concept that many of the body's problems come from blockages in the spinal nerves that serve the organs.

In short, naturopathy places great stock in the wisdom of the body to remain healthy and to heal itself.

## Aromatherapy and the Immune System

Aromatherapy is a practice dating all the way back to ancient Egypt and Greece. It uses essential oils (essences) from plants to enhance the health of the body, mind, and emotions. Aromatherapy treatments use the power of scent to raise the body's immunity to illness by calming and soothing the body, mind, and spirit. The ancients believed this restored the state of balance necessary to resist disease. Aromatherapy was practiced as a part of healing ceremonies throughout many ancient cultures. Modern aromatherapy was rediscovered in the nineteenth century by a French chemist, R.N. Gattefossé. As Gattefossé defined it, aromatherapy was "use of odiferous substances obtained from flowers, plants, and aromatic shrubs, through inhalation and application to the skin." Unknowingly, both the ancients and Gattefossé were tapping into what modern science has discovered are the psychoneuroimmunological effects of plants and flowers. Essential oils are now known to promote a balance between the sympathetic and parasympathetic nervous systems, which help relax the mind and body. In this sense, aromatherapy is a stress-reliever, stimulating the production of endorphins in the brain, which in turn rejuvenates the immune system.

> **NATURAL THERAPY VERSUS NATUROPATHY**
>
> *"The use of natural therapy does not of its own constitute naturopathy. Naturopathy involves the use of natural therapies according to certain established principles. This is where naturopathy as a science must be distinguished from folk medicine or any other natural therapy. While these techniques or tools may be employed by the naturopath, they must be used according to the basic principles of naturopathy for the end result to be naturopathic medicine."*
>
> —Dr. Ross Trattler, Better Health Through Natural Healing— How to Get Well Without Drugs or Surgery

### Essential Oils

In aromatherapy, many essential oils are believed to be imbued with specific healing properties.

- *Cardamom*—A member of the ginger family, considered a digestive aid.

- *Cedarwood*—Used in Egyptian mummification, promotes relaxation, is endowed with antifungal and antiseptic properties; fights infections of the skin and urinary tract.

- *Clary sage*—A native plant of the Mediterranean is often recommended for menstrual problems and depression.

- *Ginger*—Inhaled in China for thousands of years as a tonic to sharpen the mind and soothe the emotions, also applied to the skin to cool fevers, soothe headaches, and relieve arthritic pain.

- *Jasmine*—Believed to help with depression, anxiety, frigidity, and impotence.

- *Neroli*—A natural tranquilizer extracted from the flowers of the bitter orange tree.

- *Patchouli*—A native of the Middle East, considered a stimulant.

- *Rose*—Generally regarded as a sexual stimulant.

- *Sandalwood*—Considered to inspire tranquility.

- *Ylang-ylang*—A native flower of Malaysia and the Philippines, considered an excellent tonic for the nervous system.

Using aromatherapy is easy today. Many stores sell essential oils and a carrier oil such as almond, apricot kernel, canola, jojoba, or sunflower oil. You must dilute an essential oil in the carrier oil before applying it to your body. The essential oils are potent, and should not be used alone. Essential oils are so highly concentrated—sometimes as much as one hundred times stronger than the fresh plant or dried herb—one drop of pure essential oil applied directly to the skin can cause severe irritation. Never take essential oils internally.

### Aromatherapy Bathing and Massage

A bath or massage using aromatherapy can be a relaxing, invigorating experience that acts like a tonic to your immune system.

To prepare an aromatherapy bath, add a total of six to ten drops of essential oil or oils to a bathtub of warm water.

- *Morning Immunity Bath*

  4 drops tea tree oil
  3 drops rosemary oil
  2 drops lemon oil
  1 drop ginger oil

Disperse the essential oils well in a bathtub filled with warm water. Soak in the bath for fifteen to twenty minutes.

- *Evening Immunity Bath*

  4 drops tea tree oil
  2 drops rosewood oil
  2 drops orange oil
  2 drops clary sage oil

Add the oils to a bathtub filled with warm water and blend. Soak in the bath for fifteen to twenty minutes.

- *Immune Boosting Massage Oil*

  10 drops tea tree oil
  10 drops geranium oil
  8 drops lemon oil
  6 drops myrrh oil
  5 drops elemi oil
  4 ounces carrier oil

Place the carrier oil in a clean container, add the essential oils, and blend gently. Massage the mixture over your body once or twice daily.

## Western Strategies to Boost the Immune System

The leading edge of conventional Western medicine is adding to our knowledge of the immune system and how to ensure its optimum functioning. As more is discovered about killer cells, antibodies, and free radicals, many researchers and physicians find themselves echoing alternative medicine's recommendation. Those who want to stay healthy or get healthy must take proactive steps to improve their immune system through nutrition, exercise, and stress reduction techniques. Below are some suggestions from Western medical authorities what you can do to protect your immune system so it can function properly and keep you healthy.

### CAUTIONS WITH ESSENTIAL OILS

*According to Roberta Wilson, author of* Aromatherapy for Vibrant Health & Beauty, *people with asthma, cancer, epilepsy, high or low blood pressure, and pregnant women should be cautious about using aromatherapy. Certain essential oils can trigger asthma attacks or epileptic seizures, cause harm to cancer patients, or elevate or depress blood pressure. If you have any of the conditions listed, she suggests that you consult with a health care professional before using any essential oils.*

*Essential oils can also counteract or diminish the effectiveness of homeopathic remedies. Before beginning aromatherapy or homeopathy, check with a homeopathic physician.*

*Avoid Stress*

Not surprisingly, the first recommendation is stress must be avoided or moderated as much as possible. The neurochemicals stress produced in the brain have a direct affect on the functioning of the endocrine system and are recognized as a major factor in weakening the immune system. Those neurochemicals actually depress the body's defense systems. Much research has shown that people suffering from chronic or intense stress have weaker immune systems and frequently become ill.

*Use Antioxidant Supplements*

Current research shows vitamins and minerals act as powerful antioxidants. Many Western physicians now recommend them as powerful supplements that fight free radicals. One such dietary regime suggests:

- Beta-carotene: 25,000 IU (15 mg) per day. Beta-carotene is a precursor of vitamin A.

- Selenium: 100 to 200 mcg per day. Selenium works well with vitamin E, and taking the two together with a meal is

VITAMIN C IN FOODS

| Food Source | Vitamin C in milligrams |
| --- | --- |
| Broccoli, raw, half a cup, boiled | 49 |
| Canned grapefruit juice, 8 oz. | 72 |
| Cranberry juice cocktail, 8 oz. bottled | 108 |
| Fresh acerola juice, 8 oz. | 3,870 |
| Fresh grapefruit juice, 8 oz. | 94 |
| Fresh lemon juice, 8 oz. | 112 |
| Fresh orange juice, 8 oz. | 124 |
| Strawberries, 1 cup raw | 85 |

*"The amount of antioxidants that you maintain in your body is directly proportional to how long you will live"*

*—Dr. Richard Cutler, Director of the Antiaging Research Department at the National Institutes of Health.*

a good combination. Selenium and vitamin C interfere with each other's efficiency. Take selenium at least 30 minutes before or after taking vitamin C.

- Vitamin C: 1,000 mg two or three times per day. Calcium ascorbate soluble powder provides both vitamin C and a small amount of calcium, moreover it is non-acidic.

- Vitamin E: 400 IU once per day under age forty; twice per day over age forty. A natural source of vitamin E taken with a meal containing some fats or oils is recommended.

- Zinc picolinate: 30 mg per day.

Men require more vitamin C than women, and the doses above will vary according to your age, weight, and the amount of exercise you get.

The value of such antioxidants has been shown in a number of studies. A 1992 Canadian study found a group of elderly people given antioxidant and mineral supplements caught half as many cases of colds, flu, and infectious diseases. They also recovered from viral illnesses twice as quickly.

BETA-CAROTENE IN FOODS

| Food Source | Beta-carotene in International Units (IU) |
|---|---|
| Apricots, 3 medium sized | 2,760 |
| Broccoli, half cup, boiled | 1,090 |
| Brussels sprouts, half cup, boiled | 560 |
| Carrot, 1 raw | 20,250 |
| Carrot, half cup, sliced and boiled | 19,150 |
| Mango, 1 medium | 8,060 |
| Spinach, boiled, half cup | 7,370 |
| Sweet potato, mashed, half cup | 27,960 |

*Eat Foods High in Antioxidants*

In addition to supplements above, the right diet provides the best source of antioxidant protection. The following charts list the foods you should consider if you wish to enhance your immune system through increasing your consumption of antioxidants.

## Herbal Immune Builders

A number of herbs also appear to be natural protectors of the immune system. These include:

- *Astragalus*—Promotes production of interferon and antibodies, and increased activity of white blood cells. Prepared from the nontoxic root of a Chinese plant, *Astragalus membranaceous,* it is sold in health food stores under the name huangqi.

- *Garlic*—Increases the numbers of killer cells that protect the body against cancer. Use fresh garlic when possible.

VITAMIN E IN FOODS

| Food Source | Vitamin E in International Units (IU) |
|---|---|
| Almonds, whole, 1 oz. (28 grams) | 10.10 |
| Corn oil, 1 tablespoon | 1.90 |
| Mayonnaise, 1 tablespoon | 11.00 |
| Safflower oil, 1 tablespoon | 4.60 |
| Sunflower oil, 1 tablespoon | 6.10 |
| Sunflower seeds, dried, 1 oz. (28 g) | 14.18 |
| Wheat germ oil, 1 tablespoon | 20.30 |
| Wheat germ, dry, one third cup | 6.00 |

• *Siberian ginseng*—Protects from the harmful effects of stress.

## Chapter Recap

• The immune system is a complex system of warriors and messengers that coordinate defense against invaders throughout the entire body.

• The body can be attacked by bacteria or viruses, and by free radicals that damage cells.

• Ayurveda and Chinese medicine consider enhancing disease resistance the same as taking proactive steps to preserve your vitality and vigor.

• In Ayurveda, sexual depletion indicates low disease resistance. Rejuvenating herbs are recommended.

• Naturopathy is a method of curing disease by releasing inner vitality and allowing the body to heal itself.

- To protect the immune system, nutritional experts recommend a variety of supplements on a daily basis. These supplements act as antioxidants to scavenge free radicals and eliminate them from the body.

- For herbal immunity boosters try garlic, Siberian ginseng, and astragalus.

- Many aromatherapy blends can enhance your immune system by soothing and calming the mind.

- Many foods contain natural antioxidants.

*Recommended Reading*

Cooper, Kenneth H., M.D. *Dr. Kenneth Cooper's Antioxidant Revolution.* Nashville: Thomas Nelson Publishers, 1994.

Lin, David J. *Free Radicals and Disease Prevention, What You Must Know.* New Canaan, CT: Keats Publishing Inc., 1993.

Hurley, Judith Benn. *The Good Herb.* (New York: William Morrow and Company, Inc., 1995).

# The Anticancer and Healthy Heart Lifestyle

*T*he prevention lifestyle is a way of living that wards off the two leading causes of death in much of the Western world before they can start. When you're talking about such cancer and heart disease, prevention is paramount. This chapter is devoted to looking at how alternative medicine can help us live in such a way as to greatly reduce our chances of having either.

The Anticancer and Healthy Heart Lifestyle is based upon nutrition, exercise, and stress management. It offers some workable, pleasant, and effective ways to live cancer-preventive and heart-healthy. The anticancer lifestyle checklist and the heart healthy lifestyle checklist will benefit both your entire body and your heart.

## The Anticancer Lifestyle

As we saw in Chapter 10, the unstable oxygen molecules, called free radicals, have been linked to many serious diseases, including cancer. Free radicals attack the nucleus of cells and damage the DNA, which can then lead to cell mutation, the beginning of cancer. Common sources of these attackers are the many forms of pollution in the environment. A good defense against the formation of free radicals is the anticancer lifestyle.

### The Anticancer Lifestyle Checklist

If you wish to reduce the risk of cancer, alternative medicine recommends incorporating the following into your life:

- Eat a healthy diet, along with vitamin and mineral supplements, that contain adequate levels of antioxidants to protect your immune system and guard against cancer.

- Exercise at least thirty minutes a day. Try to maintain your ideal weight through nutrition and exercise.

- Avoid carcinogens in foods, chemicals, and the environment.

- Use alcohol in moderation. No more than four drinks a week.

- Do not smoke cigarettes, cigars, pipes, or marijuana. Avoid chewing tobacco and snuff.

- Use sunblock, hats, clothing, and other means of protection to shield yourself against ultraviolet light from the sun, a leading cause of skin cancer. But, don't let sunblock lull you into a false sense of security. Use caution between 11:00 a.m. and 3:00 p.m. when the sun's ultraviolet rays are at their most potent.

- Learn to handle or moderate stress in your life. Use meditation, progressive relaxation, or deep-breathing, aromatherapy, or any of the techniques previously suggested for soothing your mind and calming your spirit.

- Make sure your home is free of cancer causing agents such as radon, asbestos, and pesticide. Radon is an invisible gas that rises out of certain geological formations. You can check a geological map at your city or county health office to see if your house is at risk. If you are at risk, test kits can measure the amount of radon present, and there are remedial steps you can take to protect yourself.

*"I believe the doctor of the future will be a teacher as well as a physician. His or her real job will be to teach people to be healthy. Doctors will be even busier than they are now because it is a lot harder to keep people well than it is just to get them over a sickness."*
—*Dr. D. C. Jarvis,*
Folk Medicine

### The Body's Detox System

Your body is equipped with an exquisite detoxification system. It is a little known or appreciated defense system for disposing of toxic substances. For millennia, it enabled our ancestors to eat plants safely, letting nutrients through and blocking less desirable compounds. Today, it turns aside assaults from carcinogens like pollutants, pesticides, food contaminants, and industrial chemicals. How well this body's detox system works strongly influences how well you resist cancer.

### The Anticancer Diet

Avoiding cancer is a matter not only of what you avoid in your life but of what you include. Not more than twenty-five years ago, it was heresy to suggest among Western physicians that the likelihood of contracting cancer could be reduced by proper diet. However, scientists now know that molecules of certain foods are very potent defenders against free radicals and other forces that cause cancer. These anticancer foods:

- Capture and kill free radical oxygen molecules that promote cellular damage and cancer.

- Interfere with messengers that accidentally switch on oncogenes in the cell nucleus to start and encourage the cancer process.

- Neutralize other agents that activate carcinogens in the body.

- Stimulate other food enzymes to setup systems for flushing carcinogens from the body.

Cabbage and its cousins have been shown to be among the most potent anticancer foods. Adding cruciferous vegetables like cabbage (see anticancer vegetables, Chapter 1) to your menu can win you a healthy amount of chemoprevention when it comes to building a biological fortress against cancer. Studies show that a serving of cabbage once a week can slice your chances of colon

*". . . While cigarette smoking is the single most important known cause of cancer and other chronic diseases, about 70 percent of cancer isn't generally linked to smoking. Among the other factors that probably are contributing to the increased incidence of cancer, a prime candidate must be excessive free radical exposure due to the pollution of our environment. A link may also exist between free radical damage and stress."*

—*Kenneth H. Cooper, M.D.,*
Antioxidant Revolution

cancer by 66 percent. The same can be said of foods like broccoli, Brussels sprouts, and sauerkraut.

Cabbage contains helpful chemicals called dithiolthiones, that influence the enzymes that crank up the body's detoxification system by causing it to release a burst of molecules that can engage and destroy toxins, including carcinogens. Revealing the manner in which medical researchers are becoming increasingly impressed with the anticancer properties of the lowly cabbage and its cousins, Dr. Thomas Kensler of Johns Hopkins University says, "Dithiolthiones are as potent an anticancer agent as we have ever looked at. It's quite dramatic."

*Your Cancer Prevention Menu*

Start by including these vegetables in your diet: broccoli, Brussels sprouts, cabbage, cauliflower, cress, horseradish, kale, kohlrabi, mustard, radishes, rutabagas, and turnips. Then add some vegetables rich in carotenes: apricots, carrots, kale, lettuce, spinach, squash, sweet potatoes, and tomatoes. It's a case of good eating leads to good health.

In terms of how much to eat and when, follow these guidelines:

- Avoid charred meat, and salt cured, nitrate cured, and smoked foods.

- Consume 25 grams or more of dietary fiber per day.

- Eat five to nine servings of fruits and vegetables daily.

- Eat foods rich in vitamins C and E, carotenes, and selenium.

- Keep your intake of dietary fat to no more than 20 percent of total daily calories.

- Maintain your ideal weight.

## Keeping a Merry Heart

Sudden cardiac death is the leading cause of mortality in the industrialized world. Until recently, most Western medicine has treated this condition through drugs and surgery. Alternative medicine has long offered ways to prevent and reduce heart problems through natural means such as exercise, diet, and stress management. Increasingly, Western practitioners are seeing the wisdom of working with patients this way, too.

As Dr. Dean Ornish notes, coronary heart disease is largely a disease of excess, meaning that heart disease arises from exposure to a lifestyle containing excessive levels of stress and a diet containing excessive amounts of animal products. These excesses activate a web of bodily mechanisms that reduce coronary blood flow and lead to such manifestations of coronary heart disease as chest pain (angina), heart attack, or sudden cardiac failure and death.

### Heart Healthy Foods

The ideal diet for heart health contains whole grains, fresh vegetables, fruits, cooked legumes, about a tablespoon of oil per day, and nonfat yogurt (plain). Then in descending order, you can add:

- Nuts and seeds in moderation, not more than 2 tbsp. per day 3 times a week

- Nonfat skim milk

- Lowfat skim milk cheeses

- Baked or broiled lean fish

- Egg whites

Less desirable—but you can indulge in them as infrequently as possible if you must—are baked or broiled chicken or turkey with the skin removed before cooking.

A heart healthy diet omits altogether such staples of the typical American diet as cream, cream cheeses, whole milk, beef, pork, fried chicken with the skin on, coconut oil and coconut, egg yolks, and salt.

The change to a heart healthy diet can be made gradually by cutting down on red meat, for instance, before completely removing it from your menu. Little by little, start choosing foods from the top of the list, rather than from the bottom.

Garlic and raw onions have been shown to be helpful in thinning the blood by reducing its tendency to clot. Hawthorn berries are also recommended. The antioxidant diet and supplements listed above help prevent not only cancer, but also heart disease. Vitamin E at 400 IU per day for adults under forty, and 800 IU per day for adults age forty and over, is a natural blood thinner, as well as a powerful antioxidant.

Folic acid, also called folate, has been shown to reduce the cholesterol deposits that narrow the blood vessels in the cardiovascular system and heart. It does this by preventing excess amounts of an amino acid, homocysteine, which occurs naturally in the blood, but leads to cholesterol buildups at higher levels. Some medical experts are even hailing folic acid, which is part of the B-complex vitamin, as the vitamin of the decade. A dose of 400 mcg per day is the RDA for folic acid.

*A Heart Healthy Lifestyle Checklist*

Keeping in mind the diet and stress management techniques already described, here are a few more musts for a healthy heart:

- Exercise. For most people, thirty minutes of aerobic exercise five or more days a week will go a long way toward keeping the cardiovascular system in shape. Check with your medical practitioner to determine the right amount of exercise for you.

- Find and maintain your heart healthy weight.

- Find and maintain your heart healthy blood pressure and cholesterol count.

- Find ways to manage stress that will work for you.

- Eat a healthy heart diet.

## Chapter Recap

- Cancer and heart disease are two of the leading killers in the Western world. You can lower your risks of both by following a prevention lifestyle.

- The prevention lifestyle includes food, exercise, and stress management.

- Compounds found in foods can capture and snuff out free radicals, neutralize agents that would activate carcinogens, and stimulate enzymes for flushing carcinogens from the body.

- An anticancer diet includes fruits and vegetables, foods rich in vitamins C and E, carotenes and selenium, and dietary fat no more than 20 percent of your total calories.

- Avoid nitrate cured, salt cured, smoked, and charred meats.

- Maintain your ideal weight.

- Coronary disease is largely a disease of excess, harmful reactions to chronic stress, and a diet based on excessive animal products.

- Folic acid has been shown to reduce the occurrence of the cholesterol deposits that narrow blood vessels.

- The prevention lifestyle benefits your entire body.

*Recommended Reading*

Winawer, Sidney J., M.D. and Moshe Shike, M.D., *Cancer Free.* New York: Simon & Schuster, 1995.

Ornish, Dean, M.D., *Stress, Diet, and Your Heart.* New York: Holt, Rinehart & Winston, 1982.

Carper, Jean. *The Food Pharmacy.* New York: Bantam, 1989.

# *Living Longer and*

# *Loving It*

*W*hether we call it life extension, longevity, or turning back your biological clock, every one of us wants a richer and fuller life. What's more, we want to continue being physically fit and mentally alert throughout our golden years, so we can enjoy all that the third trimester of life has to offer. In this chapter we will explore some of the ways that lead to a long and healthy life. Included here are the most important recommendations that alternative medicine, in partnership with conventional medicine, has to offer for extending your life and health.

## *Why We Age*

To combat aging, we need to know more about the aging process and the reasons it takes place. Unfortunately, while research into this matter continues, and there are many theories, there are as yet no definitive answers.

Theories about why we age fall into two broad groups:

- Aging and death result from random errors of nature.

- We are biologically programmed to age and die.

*IN THIS CHAPTER:*

- *The theories of how we age*

- *Why maintaining vitality is an antiaging strategy*

- *Why traditional Chinese medicine believes we can live to one hundred—and how it proposes we do it*

- *A nutritional antiaging program*

- *The importance of aerobic and muscular fitness in an antiaging program*

*"Look to this day, for it is life, the very life of life. In its brief course lie all the verities and realities of your existence: the bliss of growth, the glory of action, the splendor of beauty. For yesterday is but a dream, and tomorrow is only a vision, but this day, well lived, makes all your yesterdays a dream of happiness, and all your tomorrows a vision of hope. Look well, therefore, to this day. Such is the salutation of the dawn."*
—*From the Sanskrit*

*Aging and Death As Random Errors of Nature*

Scientists who support this theory believe that, although nature intended us to procreate and then die at some time, it was left to chance as to how and when death would occur. As a result, our body is simply reacting to various forces that create errors in your metabolism, making us prone to disease and decay. The following theories fall under this group:

- *Free radical theory*—Proposes that unstable oxygen molecules, free radicals, damage parts of the body's cells by stealing electrons and setting off chain reactions which destroy essential DNA and RNA. Some researchers consider the discovery of free radicals and their role, not only in aging, but in causing disease, as one of the most important discoveries of recent decades. This theory has much support these days and is being studied in many other experiments. Antioxidants combat free radical activity. This has lead many physicians to recommend the introduction of antioxidant nutrients into the diet, in the form of certain vegetables and nutritional supplements.

- *Immune system theory*—Proposes the immune system stops functioning in its normal fashion over time, and no longer is as efficient at acting as the body's first line of defense against harmful substances that enter the body and threaten cells. The theory rests on two major findings. With age, the level of antibodies in the body declines and many autoimmune diseases occur with age, indicating that the body loses its ability to distinguish between its own cells and foreign cells.

- *Wear and tear theory*—Proposes that the body and its cells are damaged through stress and toxins from our diet and the environment, which simply wear them down each passing year. In addition, contemporary diets slanted toward foods like fats, sugars, caffeine, and alcohol also tax and age the organs. When we are young, our body produces sufficient chemicals to combat the toxins filling us and repairs the cellular wear and tear they cause. However, as we grow older the body no longer manufactures sufficient chemicals to combat these toxins and undo cellular damage as quickly and widely. More cells are damaged than the body can restore or replace, and thus, we age and lose our resistance to infirmity and disease.

### Aging As a Biological Imperative

The second group of theories contend that aging is programmed into our genes. Aging is ingrained in our evolutionary inheritance. Its supporters believe that human beings have a biological clock that ticks down the years and knows when to set the aging process in motion. Let's look at the leading theories that contend there is a biological clock controlling aging.

- *Genetic control theory*—Proposes that our DNA is encoded with a pre-programmed set of instructions that determine how quickly we age and how long we live. However, because we are all unique individuals, there is some variation in our programs, causing some people live to age seventy-five and others to one hundred. Human DNA, which carries a vast amount of information about each and every person, determining why some of us are tall and others are short, why some are optimistic and others feel pessimistic, and why some have freckles and others don't. Proponents of this theory hold it is equally possible our genes also contain codes that determine how long we will live.

- *Neuroendocrine theory*—Proposes that the body's hormonal system is responsible for determining aging. The hypothalamus which regulates the endocrine glands in the body, controls many critical processes including growth, metabolism, energy production, cellular repair, and sexual maturity. According to this theory, as we age and reach sexual maturity, there is no reason to maintain the same level of hormonal upkeep. The hypothalamus then begins to produce less and less of its hormones and the entire endocrine/immune system slows down and ceases to function as efficiently. Recent research, for example, shows that DHEA (dehydroepiandrosterone), the hormone produced by the adrenal glands, is very high when we are born and remains high until we are about twenty-five years old. Then it begins to decline sharply so that by the time we are sixty-five, we produce only 10 percent of the amount of DHEA we produced when we were age twenty. The hypothalamus controls the adrenal glands, and it is believed the loss of DHEA is an indicator of how the hormonal and immune systems slows down.

### Waiting for the Verdict on Aging

Discovering which theory holds the key to aging will take years of research, and it may be that each theory contains some part of the truth. In fact, recent scientific research seems to support almost all the theories to some extent. It may very well be that some people die from wear and tear, others from free radicals destroying their cells and inducing cancer, and still others from a genetic code that allows them to stay on earth for as long as they are programmed to do so.

Whichever theory or combination is true, the good news is that the alternative healing traditions can help increase your chances of living a long, productive life. Through following the nutritional, physical, mental, and spiritual guidelines these traditions have to offer, you can maintain a healthy mind and body for many decades, without having to fear the debilitating illnesses that bring old age and death. As Part 1 of this book indicates, the concept of maintaining your vital life force that runs through alternative medicine gives the key to staying healthy for as long as you can.

In this sense, Parts 1 and 2 of this book are already your guide to longevity. Following their recommendations for diet, exercise, breathing, stress reduction, and building your immune system are your best guide to increasing your opportunities for a long, healthful life. The next two sections offer additional suggestions for increasing longevity and enjoying a healthy old age, drawn from alternative healing traditions.

## Traditional Chinese Medicine and Longevity

According to Taoist teachings, the human body was designed by nature to live an average of one hundred years. With the right practices of longevity, it is believed that one hundred fifty years or more are possible. One extremely long-lived man who illustrated this possibility was Lee Ching-yuen, a Taoist adept and a master herbalist, who lived to be more than one hundred years old. He ate mostly lightly steamed vegetables, fresh fruit, and tonic herbs. Among his most favored herbs were ginseng, garlic, polygonum multiflorum, and gotu kola. He also learned and regularly practiced Chi gong energy work.

### Chinese Prescriptions for Long Life

Some of the practices in traditional Chinese medicine that lead to health, vitality, and longevity include:

- *Deep breathing and exercise*—Taoists believe energy work is key to prolonging life. Deep breathing is regarded as a second heart, helping the heart circulate blood. It is also believed deep breathing strengthens the body's immunity to illness and aging by switching on the parasympathetic circuit, developing positive biofeedback between the nervous system and the endocrine system.

- *Emotional balance*—Emotional imbalance is the greatest threat to the equilibrium we need to cultivate longevity. In the Chinese view, it is impossible to maintain the healthy balance of internal energies upon which long life is based without emotional balance and mental equanimity. In fact, the older you get, the more important this equilibrium becomes to your life. Through the practice of meditation, rhythmic exercise, deep breathing, and other techniques, traditional Chinese medicine offers ways to cultivate emotional balance.

- *Fasting*—Fasting is espoused as a quick and effective method to purify the tissues, organs, and blood of the body, and to prevent premature aging. The main toxins to be concerned about are the ubiquitous pollutants in the environment. Modern laboratory experiments on animals have demonstrated periodic fasting can extend their life span up to 50 percent.

- *Mental clarity*—One of the essentials for achieving a long life is mental clarity. With a clear mind you can continue with healthful and spiritually uplifting Taoist practices, keep your head in charge of your heart, and stay on the Great Highway of Tao.

- *Nutrition*—Taoist practices eliminate all processed foods. At least 30 to 50 percent of the diet is raw fresh foods. Foods and spices are classified into cooling (yin) and warming (yang) categories and only very pure water is used for cooking and drinking.

- *Sexual power*—Taoism teaches a sexual yoga, a way of balancing and exchanging vital energy with a partner, for the purpose of increasing the sexual vitality that enhances longevity. Maintaining an active sexual life into advanced age, while practicing certain techniques that increase rather than deplete sexual vitality, benefits longevity in many ways. Among these is overriding the body's timetables for aging and obsolescence, sending it a message that you are still young and vital.

- *Supplements*—Supplements for longevity include tonic herbs noted as improving health and vitality by stimulating the organs and the blood. Modern Chinese medicine endorses the use of vitamin and mineral supplements, though natural tonics are still preferred.

## The Modern Nutritional Approach to Longevity

As you might guess, the antiaging diet is very similar to the immune boosting diet, the healthy heart diet, and the anticancer diet. Each diet helps you avoid disease and maintain your vitality, so you are effectively granted additional productive years in life by following them. Their common thread that all combat the damaging effects of free radicals, now believed to be one of the leading causes of cancer, heart disease, and aging. A defense against their damaging activities is a diet rich in antioxidants. These diets are also rich in *phytonutrients*, natural chemicals in plants that are now known, from abundant scientific studies, to be very effective preventers of disease.

People who eat abundant amounts of vegetables and fruits reduce their risk of developing cancer and heart disease by one-third to one-half. This has been demonstrated in over two hundred studies on diet and disease. Individuals who follow this nutritional regime have higher blood levels of antioxidants such as vitamins C and E, beta-carotene, other carotenes, and other antioxidants. This diet has been found to be a dependable antiaging regimen able to prolong life span and prevent certain health problems.

### Antiaging Vitamins and Minerals

Several vitamins and minerals are thought to play as strong a role in preventing aging as they do in preventing cancer and heart disease:

- *Folic acid*—One of the B vitamins, folic acid, has been called the vitamin of the decade because of its effectiveness in reducing the risk of cholesterol buildup in the arteries, heart disease, and cancer.

- *Vitamin A*—This vitamin, obtained primarily from the carotenoid nutrients that come from orange, yellow, and green vegetables and fruits, seems to have youth-enhancing and protective abilities of its own. In a 1995 Harvard study, it was confirmed that lycopene, a carotenoid found in tomatoes, reduces your risk of prostate cancer by nearly

*"When the three treasures of essence, energy, and spirit remain calm, they nourish you day by day and make you strong. When they are hyperactive, they deplete you day by day and make you old."*

—Wen Tzu Classic
(first century A.D.)

50 percent. Some researchers point out that the active ingredient, lycopene, is released in greater amounts by cooking the tomatoes to approximately 300 degrees F. This indicates that tomato sauces would be healthful, eaten three to five times a week for best effect. Beta-carotene, found abundantly in carrots and sweet potatoes, can also reduce risks of cancer. Vitamin A has also been shown to be good for vision, and may help delay or prevent age-related blindness.

- *Vitamin C*—Studies also show that by taking higher amounts of vitamin C, you are less likely to develop cataracts as you grow older. Vitamin C can provide strong protection against cancers of the mouth, esophagus, stomach, and pancreas, and appears to lower the risk of lung, breast, cervical, and rectal cancers.

- *Vitamin D, calcium, and magnesium*—Sufficient amounts of calcium and vitamin D (they work together) can reduce your risk of osteoporosis, a bone thinning disease associated with aging. The calcium strengthens your bones, while the vitamin D increases the absorption and deposition of the calcium. Sadly, studies show that women who are particularly at risk, generally get only half the calcium they need in their diets. Magnesium is often combined with calcium in supplements. It has a role in preventing osteoporosis, lowering blood pressure, and regulating heartbeats.

- *Vitamin E*—In two Harvard University studies, participants taking 100 IU of vitamin E every day had a 50 percent lower risk of heart disease. The United States Department of Agriculture Human Nutrition Research Center on Aging found that 200 IU of vitamin E increased immunity in elderly people, reduced muscle damage from exercise, and slowed the progress of Alzheimer's disease. Cancer studies reveal that keeping up higher levels of vitamin E can reduce the risk of tumor development, and cancer of the lung, stomach, colon, and sex organs.

• Zinc picolinate—Medical experts recommend taking 30 mg of zinc picolinate daily to enhance the immune system, fight infections, and act as an antioxidant.

## Maintaining Your Youth through Sports and Fitness

It cannot be emphasized enough that, other than nutrition, maintaining your physical fitness is crucial to keeping your biological age younger than your chronological age. In fact, the importance of fitness is no longer a principle of alternative health alone. Even conventional Western medicine has now accepted fitness into the mainstream of antiaging and wellness ideas. Research has shown the value of physical fitness does not derive simply from the building of muscles or the deep breathing, but from the effects both of these have on all body systems. In short, exercise is a holistic wellness activity, improving many aspects of your mind and body.

### Becoming Aerobically Fit

Many types of exercise increase aerobic fitness, improving the way your

---

**DR. LINUS PAULING'S REGIMEN FOR BETTER HEALTH & LONGEVITY**

*According to the famed Dr. Linus Pauling, your longevity regimen should incorporate the following guidelines:*

• *Alcohol—Consume in moderation.*
• *Cigarettes—Do not use.*
• *Exercise—Exercise daily. However, do not at any time exert yourself physically beyond your normal capabilities.*
• *Mineral supplements—One mineral supplement daily, such as one tablet of Bronson Vitamin-mineral formula, which provides 100 mg of calcium, 18 mg of iron, 0.15 mg of iodine, 1 mg of copper, 25 mg of magnesium, 3 mg of manganese, 15 mg of zinc, 0.015 mg of molybdenum, 0.015 mg of chromium, and 0.015 mg of selenium.*
• *Stress—Avoid it. Work at a job you like. Be happy with your family.*
• *Sugar—Fifty pounds or less yearly (sucrose, raw sugar, brown sugar, honey), which is half the present U.S. average. Do not add sugar to tea or coffee. Do not eat high sugar foods. Avoid sweet desserts. Do not drink soft drinks.*
• *Super-B tablets—Take one or two every day to provide good amounts of the B vitamins.*
• *Vegetables and fruit—Eat some daily.*
• *Vitamin A—25,000 IU tablet daily.*
• *Vitamin C—6 grams to 18 grams (which translates into 6,000 to 18,000 mg), or more daily.*
• *Vitamin E—400 IU, 800 IU, or 1600 IU daily.*
• *Water—Drink a minimum of six glasses daily.*

lungs and cardiovascular system deliver oxygen to your muscles. Research demonstrates that aerobic exercise benefits the entire body. It helps the heart become stronger, so even when resting, it can beat at a slower rate. It improves the flow of blood throughout your body and tones your muscles, especially in your legs, which in turn helps your circulation return blood to the heart. This in turn helps the heart work less when pumping blood back through the veins, reducing the risk of stroke. The improved circulation also removes fatty deposits in the arteries, which further lessens your risk of heart attack and stroke.

The benefits of aerobic exercise on various systems of the body are very intertwined, so improvements in one bodily system, like the muscles, trigger improvements in others, like the heart. Ultimately, aerobic exercise can be thought of as benefiting the heart, the circulatory system, the lungs, the blood, and the body's complex hormonal system all at once! You simply can't beat aerobic exercise for the contribution it makes to longevity.

Medical experts agree you have the power to change your aerobic fitness for better or for worse. If you don't exercise aerobically, you will lose your natural aerobic fitness. By the time they turn sixty-five, men and women who do not exercise will have aerobic fitness 40 percent lower than that of young adults.

If you aren't currently performing any aerobic exercise, it's never too late to begin. Start with brisk walking, running, or cycling. Go swimming or cross-country skiing if you have the opportunity.

### Building Muscle

Building muscle also benefits your entire body in multitudinous ways. First, muscle is active tissue that burns calories both at rest and during exercise. Fat doesn't. The less muscle you have, the easier it is to become overweight and maintain high levels of body fat that clog your arteries and tax the heart. This heightens the risk of stroke and certain types of cancers. It is natural for body fat to increase as you grow older. The bodies of men at age twenty-five average about 18 percent fat, but by age sixty-five, fat averages about 38 percent. You can change this by keeping the fat ratio down through a muscle building regime, whatever your current age.

Furthermore, muscle building is a critical corollary to aerobic fitness. In most aerobic programs, you are exercising primarily your legs and the muscles that lie below your waist. However, two-thirds of the body's muscle mass is above the waist. By starting a muscle building program that exercises the upper body, you improve your overall fitness by two-thirds. Upper-body and muscle-building programs also ward off such chronic infirmities of old age as weakness in legs, back problems, and inflammations of joints and ligaments.

### WRITE YOUR GOALS FOR REJUVENATION

*Dr. Deepak Chopra has written, "We program our consciousness to a set span of aging, and our biology responds to that programming." Many people have wrongly accepted what they believe is an inevitable decline that accompanies aging. But Dr. Chopra points to the need to throw out such outmoded concepts of aging, and reprogram our consciousness to keep us younger and healthier.*

*Setting these goals down in writing can be a powerful tool for programming our unconscious in such a way as to bring them about. Not only will you feel more committed by seeing your goals in black and white, but you will find that reviewing your goals , whenever you feel your motivation waning, can be an effective method of renewing your commitment.*

### *Whole Body Exercise*

Ultimately, most medical experts recommend a combination of aerobic and muscle-building exercise. One ideal form is cross country skiing, also called Nordic skiing. Following trails through a forest, you not only ski down the hills, you also climb up them. It's great exercise for the heart and lungs, and muscle groups throughout the body, including the abdominal muscles, chest, back, triceps, thighs, and buttocks.

If you live in a warmer climate you might try a brisk game of tennis, and different kinds of cycling, including mountain biking. Finally there's weight-lifting and flexibility exercises. It's safest to begin under the guidance of a trainer or as part of a group at a gym. Consult with your medical practitioner for guidelines before undertaking any strenuous exercise regime.

## Chapter Recap

- Some theories suggest we age and die due to normal wear and tear, or that our immune system breaks down, or that free radicals damage our cells and our DNA.

- Other theories suggest we live according to a biological clock in our genes that cannot be changed.

- The way to ensure a long, productive, healthy life is to maintain your vitality, as many alternative therapies recommend.

- Traditional Chinese medicine regards longevity as the greatest prize for health seekers, and helps them toward it through nutrition, supplements, fasting, environmental factors, exercises, sexual discipline, clarity, and emotional balance.

- Contemporary medical approaches to longevity is based on foods rich in chemicals called antioxidants that can counter the aging effects of free radical damage and supply us with protective phytonutrients.

- The sports/fitness approach to longevity combines aerobic fitness and muscle-building to benefit all the systems of the body, reducing the risk of diseases such as stroke, high blood pressure, heart disease, and cancer, and the degenerative conditions traditionally connected with aging.

### Recommended Reading

Arnott, Robert, M.D. *Dr. Bob Arnott's Guide to Turning Back the Clock*. Boston: Little, Brown and Company, 1995.

Reid, Daniel. *The Complete Book of Chinese Health and Healing*. Boston MA: Shambala, 1995.

Yang, Jwing-ming. *The Root of Chinese Chi Kung*. New York: YMAA, 1988.

Reid, Daniel. *The Tao of Health, Sex and Longevity*. New York: Simon & Schuster, 1989.

Cleary, Thomas. *Vitality, Energy, Spirit*. Boston: Shambala, 1992.

# *Healing Therapies and*

# *Treatable Ailments*

In the previous parts of this book, you discovered how to maintain and rejuvenate your vitality, how to understand the mind/body connection that influences so many aspects of your health, and how to live a prevention lifestyle that leads to longevity, health, and happiness.

Part 4 is dedicated to a consumer's survey of the leading alternative healing traditions, and the treatments they recommend for some of our most common physical illnesses and complaints. First, you'll be taken on a tour of twenty-five leading alternative medical traditions, each with its own precepts and approaches to health and healing. You will learn how these traditions can help heal twenty-five of the ailments people ask about most, from the common cold to ear infections, indigestion, and obesity.

With this knowledge, you'll be able to determine whether the next time you are ill, an alternative therapy might provide an alternative or addition to traditional Western treatment. In time, you won't even notice which type of healing tradition you choose from, as you move toward a more integrated approach to health that utilizes the best of all traditions—conventional Western and alternative.

# A Guide to the Leading

# Alternative Therapies

*T*hough they may share ideas and even practices, all alternative therapies are not alike. They have many differences in philosophy and approach. Some alternative health traditions work better for some people, different traditions seem to prove more beneficial for other people.

This chapter evaluates twenty-five leading alternative healing traditions in terms of:

- Usefulness as a form of healing

- Research findings about its efficacy from the most recent scientific journals

- Practitioners of note

- Comparisons with Western medicine and other traditions

- Conditions and illnesses proved most beneficial from healing

The most important characteristic all the differing traditions share is the belief that the body has natural healing powers of its own which can throw off illness if aided properly. All alternative medical traditions also share the following five approaches to treating illness and promoting health:

- Dietary modification, including foods to take or avoid

- Environmental modifications, including elimination of toxins or changes to surroundings

- Herbal treatments, including the use of natural tonics, herbs, and specific vitamin and mineral supplements

- Mind/body (psychological) modifications, including stress reduction and meditation

- Modifications of the physical body, including movement and exercise

Because they rely on the body's natural healing abilities, some alternative approaches to wellness take time. The body can't regain its balance and marshal its natural forces overnight. Complete healing may take weeks or even months, but the healing can be long lasting and comprehensive.

## Acupuncture

Acupuncture probably dates back four thousand years or more. While Western doctors use specific surface pressure points for diagnosis, acupuncturists use them for treatment as well. Acupuncture is based on the principle that our vital energy is distributed to various points on the body, and illness results when these points become blocked. These points are believed to link the nerves between the skin surface and internal organs. Acupuncture liberates blocked energy and restores health by inserting probes into these acupuncture points and opening them up again.

Select an acupuncturist with care and get a recommendation, if possible. A practitioner of acupuncture needs skill to place the needles so as to open the flow without causing pain. Absolute sterilization of needles is essential, and the best acupuncturists use individually wrapped disposable needles that are discarded after one use.

*An Electronic Model*

Studies of acupuncture points have revealed they have electrical properties. Acupuncture points may be something like the printed circuits in microprocessors and other electronic devices that control so much of modern technology. One principle of electronics is that very small changes in electrical flow can produce very large results. It only takes one-tenth of one volt, positive or negative, to turn on a tiny transistor. The voltage is so small only sophisticated digital meters can detect it. That transistor turned on using a printed circuit board could signal a huge two-ton alternator to turn on, generating over twelve hundred volts. Acupuncture may work because the metal probe the practitioner uses conducts the electricity existing in the cells which alters their electrical field. The amounts are as insignificant as those in a transistor, but they can produce much larger results in the human body.

*Usefulness*—Acupuncture is used to treat a wide range of complaints, both mental and physical (over one hundred according to the World Health Organization). Success in relieving addictions ranging from heroin addiction to the more common alcohol and cigarette addictions has been credited to acupuncture. It has also demonstrated value as an anesthesic during surgery.

*Research*—At the Beijing Neurosurgical Institute, the majority of neck and head surgeons use acupuncture as the preferred means of anesthesia and pain relief. A UCLA study determined that acupuncture reduced migraine and muscle tension headaches in frequency and severity. Other research has provided evidence that acupuncture is a viable alternative to analgesic (pain-killing) drugs. Addicts in addiction recovery programs who were also treated with acupuncture were 50 percent more likely to remain drug free than those in the same programs who did not receive acupuncture.

An article by A. Chen, M.D., in the *American Journal of Acupuncture*, described "Effective Acupuncture Therapy for Migraine: Review and Comparison of Prescriptions with Recommendations for Improved Results." *The American Journal of*

*Acupuncture* published the results of a study by G. S. Chen on "The Effect of Acupuncture Treatment on Carpal Tunnel Syndrome."

*Practitioners*—Acupuncture is available from licensed health professionals, including physicians, and others with acupuncture training who are licensed to perform this therapy. The credential is generally indicated by the designation of L.Ac. Acupuncture is practiced worldwide, but is considered a conventional therapy in Asia and an alternative therapy in the West.

*Comparisons*—With its emphasis on gently opening the body's blocked energy, acupuncture can be compared to acupressure. This is also a non-invasive therapy that works to restart blocked energy by applying touch to acupuncture points. As an analgesic, acupuncture compares to aspirin and other conventional pain medications.

*Conditions or illnesses best suited for*—Acupuncture is a therapy of choice for those suffering from chronic pain like arthritis, where it compares favorably in many ways with the effects of conventional medical and surgical analgesics.

## Alexander Technique

The Alexander Technique was developed in the early 1900s by F. Mathias Alexander, an Australian actor who performed dramatic monologues from the plays of William Shakespeare. Alexander found himself constantly losing his voice in the middle of a performance. When he consulted physicians, they told him to get plenty of rest, which for him offered only temporary relief. During the period from about 1890 to 1900, the actor carefully observed himself in front of a three-part mirror. He observed that he lost his voice when he distorted his head and neck in his habitual way, with his head and neck slumped downward, compressing the larynx and causing him to strain to get his breath. By realigning his head, neck, and torso in better ways, Alexander's voice returned to its former strength. Additional observations convinced him that proper alignment of the head, neck, and spine produced therapeutic benefits for his overall physical, mental, and emotional functioning. From these experiments, Alexander developed the technique of reeducating the body that forms the basis of the Alexander Technique.

The goal of the Alexander Technique is not only healing treatment, but an entire physical self-reeducation process guided by an expert teacher. It points to a comprehensive integration of mind and body by retraining people to realign and balance their moves and postures. Clients learn to eliminate patterns that interfere with the optimal performance or function of the body.

Therapy is performed by teachers of the Alexander Technique, who received training under the guidance of the Society of Teachers of the Alexander Technique. Each session has two goals: first to help the client find different ways of moving that are easier and more efficient, thus reducing wear and tear on body structure and internal organs, second to help the client detect and let go of excessive tension that has been held unconsciously in the body.

*Usefulness*—Benefits of the Alexander Technique include a significant lowering of physical and mental stress, improved breathing, and relief for conditions ranging from arthritis, back pain, and breathing disorders to stress related diseases.

*Research*—A Tufts University study found that those trained through the Alexander Technique were successful in unlearning physical habits that interfere with or impair normal physical balance.

*Practitioners*—The Society of Teachers of the Alexander Technique, and schools for training teachers are in Europe and North America. The curriculum is based on research and practice by the founder of the Alexander Technique, F. Mathias Alexander, and on current knowledge of body mechanics, posture, physiology, and movement.

*Conditions or illnesses best suited for*—It helps release tensions held unconsciously in the body, and reeducate patients to stand, sit, and move in ways that are harmonious and more efficient. Many artists have studied this technique and found it honed the creative skills. The Alexander Technique is taught at some of the world's leading schools of dramatic arts. The noted educator John Dewey considered the technique to be so beneficial to learning and well-being that he recommended it be taught in the elementary school curriculum.

## Aromatherapy and Essential Oils

Aromatherapy uses naturally distilled essences of plants to promote positive changes in physical, mental, and emotional health. The essences, called essential oils, can be purchased in many health food stores, and are intended to restore balance and harmony.

The term aromatherapy can be misleading. The effect of the oils is pharmacological as well as aromatic, in that they can also be absorbed into body tissues to carry out their role in healing. Aromatherapy can be used as self care, for both health and cosmetic reasons.

Aromatherapy dates back to antiquity, but the contemporary version was popularized by a nineteenth century French chemist and perfumer, R. M. Gattefossé, whose studies helped to revive the ancient art. Working in his laboratory one day, Gattefossé burned his hand. For relief he plunged it into the nearest container of liquid, which turned out to be lavender oil. The rapid and complete healing of his burns led him to explore the therapeutic uses of other essential oils from plants and flowers.

Practitioners say that aromatherapy, by gently activating the body's own healing energies, helps to restore balance to body, mind, and spirit. Aromatherapy may tap into the pyschoneuroimmunological communication in the brain to produce neurotransmitters that soothe and calm us. Aromatherapy works on the olfactory sensors in the brain. They have direct connections with the hypothalamus which controls the hormonal and immune systems.

Some one hundred and fifty to three hundred or more essential oils are available worldwide. Books available in health food stores can tell you about all the most popular essences and supply directions on exactly how to use them, at what strength, and at what dilution. The diluted essences can be dabbed on the skin, inhaled, or absorbed in bath water, depending on the specific directions.

To use aromatherapy effectively, you will need to consult a qualified aromatherapist, or take advantage of guidebooks that list the oils, along with their medicinal and beauty benefits, their emotional effects, primary actions, and cautions. The formulas for aromatherapy blends are given, with the proper dilutions, and should be heeded, because essential oils need to be diluted in carrier oil before use to avoid harmful effects.

*Guidelines*—When using essential oils, always follow these simple guidelines for the most beneficial result:

- Always dilute essential oils in a carrier oil.

- Follow directions for blending carefully. You can use fewer, but not more drops of the essential oil than directions usually give.

- For children and infants, dilute even more.

- If the smell of an essential oil displeases you, don't use it. Learn to trust your senses.

- Inhale essential oils only for short periods of time.

- Keep bottles tightly capped and away from sunlight and heat.

- Use only glass containers in which to store and pour the oils.

- Use only pure essential oils, not synthetics.

- When in doubt about how to use an essential oil, check with a qualified aromatherapist or health professional.

*Usefulness*—Aromatherapy is useful for the alleviation of a wide range of health problems, from arthritis to yeast infections, and for therapy of the skin and hair. Skin specialists and cosmetologists find aromatherapy can enhance the health of skin and hair. In addition, it soothes and relaxes both mind and body. Because stress is considered the root cause of many major illnesses, this may be aromatherapy's greatest service.

*Research*—Much of the research on aromatherapy has been conducted in Europe, where the therapy is widely used. The *British Medical Journal* published a paper on "Treating Irritable Bowel Syndrome with Peppermint Oil." *The Journal of the American Pharmaceutical Association* published research on "The In Vitro Antibacterial Activity of Essential Oils and Oil Combinations," and "Antibacterial Activity of Essential Oil Vapors." *Aromatherapy Quarterly* published "Brain Research and Essential Oils." *The Journal of Psychophysiology* published research on "The Effects of Low Concentration Odors on EEG Activity and Behavior." In addition to professional journals there are nearly one hundred books that concern aromatherapy.

*Practitioners*—There are many aromatherapists at work today. Massage therapists and other alternative therapists also make use of the healing power of scent. Warning: Currently, aromatherapists are not licensed. Be sure you are working with a knowledgeable practitioner and observe the precautions for diluting the essential oils given above.

*Comparisons*—Aromatherapy can be compared for its benefits to skin and hair to some of the conventional treatments of dermatology. Its effects on stress management can be compared to the relaxing and mood-modifying properties of certain types of drugs and of exercise. Its effects on alleviating health problems are used in homeopathy, naturopathy, and nutritional medicine.

*Conditions or illnesses best suited for*—Stress-related conditions, relaxation, sexual stagnation, and loss of desire. Aromatherapy oils and blends are also ideal for their skin, hair, and beauty benefits.

Specific health problems can also be alleviated by application of aromatherapy following known formulas and guidelines.

## Ayurvedic Medicine

Ayurveda, a holistic system of health and longevity that arose in India is likely the world's oldest system of natural medicine. It is believed to be the source of Egyptian, Chinese, Greek, and Persian medicine. The name comes from *veda* meaning knowledge or science, and *ayus* meaning life or life span, combining to mean science of life or knowledge of life span. Ayurveda practices preventive medicine, promoting wellness by steadily building mental, emotional, and physical strength. Ayurveda is truly holistic in that it sees the person as an integrated whole, rather than a collection of body parts and organs requiring specialized attention. Ayurveda studies the mental, physical, emotional, and spiritual sides of the person before reaching a diagnosis.

Ayurveda divides all humans into ten different mind and body types, reflecting their physical and emotional characteristics. In Ayurveda, knowing your body type is an important prerequisite for therapy, as all recommendations for exercise, diet, and other treatments are directed toward these ten specific mind/body makeups. Body types are basically described as vata, pitta, and kapha or a combination of these three. They are described in a chart in Chapter 1. To determine your dosha or body type, there are also a series of written tests you can take in *Boundless Energy, The Complete Mind/Body Program for Overcoming Chronic Fatigue* by Deepak Chopra, M.D.

After your body type is determined, Ayurvedic therapy will advise adjustments to your diet, stress management, exercise, lifestyle changes, and herbal treatments to balance your body correctly for its type. Reported benefits of Ayurveda include increased physical health and inner peace. While many elements of Ayurveda appear exotic and strange, especially at first, in India it is thought of as a system of natural health and healing that deals with the day-to-day needs of the body, mind, and spirit. These basic needs are met in unique ways through familiar channels:

- *Breathing*—A discipline of deep and conscious breathing—*pranayama*—can improve health, relieve stress, and aid meditation.

- *Vegetarian food*—Suited to your unique body type or dosha. Unhealthy foods for your dosha are eliminated from the diet altogether.

- *Exercise*—Yoga disciplines of stretching and postures aid in neurorespiratory and neuromuscular integration.

- *Meditation*—This discipline of expectant listening allows you to seek and find guidance for body, mind, and spirit.

- *Herbal medicine*—The tradition of using natural plant products for healing, tonics, and rejuvenation is honored in both Western and Chinese medicine as well as Ayurveda. The extensive inventory of herbal treatments in Ayurvedic medicine works with breathing, food, exercise, and meditation in a system directed toward prevention of disease, as well as healing when needed.

*Usefulness*—As a complete system of natural healing, Ayurveda is applicable to a range of health conditions, maintaining the body, mind, and spirit in a condition that prevents the onset of disease.

*Research*—*The Journal of the American Medical Association* published an article by D. Chopra, H.M. Sharma, and B.D. Triguna on the subject of "Maharishi Ayurveda: Modern Insights into Ancient Medicine." Deepak Chopra, M.D., has explained the theory and practice of Ayurvedic medicine in his book *Boundless Energy*, and in other articles and publications on the subject.

*Practitioners*—Ayurveda is practiced by Ayurvedic physicians. Some Western trained medical doctors, such as Deepak Chopra, integrate Ayurveda into their practice, writing, and teaching. Ayurvedic remedies and exercises available for self care are also available through books.

*Comparisons*—Ayurveda, with its use of diet, herbs, and exercise, can be compared to traditional Chinese medicine.

*Conditions or illnesses best suited for*—The aim of Ayurveda is to balance and tone the body, mind, and spirit so disease does not occur in the first place. If health conditions or ailments arise, then Ayurveda uses diet, herbal supplements, and exercise treatments according to its principles and practice.

## Bach Remedies

Bach Remedies are floral preparations developed by Dr. Edward Bach, a bacteriologist who worked in several London hospitals and died in 1936. He devised approximately thirty-eight flower remedies based on diluted solutions of the flower's substances, brewed by letting the flowers soak in water in direct sunlight for a period. This floral solution is then taken by the patient. These floral remedies are mostly aimed at curing emotional states rather than physical conditions, but Dr. Bach also devised a combination of five remedies which he called the Rescue Remedy, and prescribed as a comprehensive cure for stress, trauma, and other emotional difficulties. Bach remedies, including the Rescue Remedy, are available in many holistic pharmacies and health food stores.

*Usefulness*—Help in alleviating stress, trauma, and emotional upsets.

*Research*—In a study at the Bellevue Medical Center of New York University, researchers found that 80 percent of patients treated with flower remedies showed improvements in their health. In about 20 percent who showed no physical improvement showed significant emotional improvement.

*Practitioners*—Anyone. Bach remedies are available in health food stores for use as self care.

*Comparisons*—Using the essences of flowers and other plant parts for emotional and physical health can be compared to aromatherapy, and to a certain degree, to herbal medicine, and to homeopathy.

*Conditions or illnesses best suited for*—Emotional conditions like stress, depression, fear, and anger.

## Biofeedback Training

Biofeedback is a method of gaining conscious control over many bodily reactions involved in creating wellness by monitoring your own emotional state with specially designed equipment. Biofeedback training typically links a person with an electrical monitoring device that gives them feedback on one of the body's vital functions. An example is the heart rate monitor, clipped on to the end of the finger. Every time your pulse beats, the monitor beeps, and there is a flash of a light. Eventually you learn how to alter and slow the pulse, which is vital for those challenged by stress and heart disease.

Proponents of biofeedback point to its success in treating those with emotionally based problems. There is also evidence biofeedback can benefit people seeking relief from problems of the digestive, heart, and nervous systems. Migraine headaches and sleeplessness have also been successfully treated with biofeedback.

In the area of mind/body medicine, biofeedback is an ideal adjunct to meditation, imagery, and visualization techniques.

*Usefulness*—Biofeedback training had been useful for stress management, pain relief, stomach problems, cardiopulmonary disease, fatigue, asthma, insomnia, headache, and muscular problems.

*Research*—A recent article in the journal, *Primary Care: Clinics in Office Practice,* "Hypertension and Biofeedback" reported that biofeedback helped people successfully learn to take more control over their body functions, such as relaxation, and the regulation of blood pressure. Dr. David Shapiro of Harvard Medical School uses biofeedback to help patients control their high blood pressure.

Biofeedback's effectiveness in relieving the pain of headaches has been confirmed in studies at the famous Menninger Clinic.

The *Proceedings of the National Academy of Sciences of the United States* published "Behavioral Method for the Treatment of Idiopathic Scoliosis." *Biofeedback and Self Regulation* published a study on "Fifteen-Month Follow-Up with Asthmatics Utilizing EMG/Incentive Inspirometer Feedback."

*Comparisons*—Biofeedback training can be compared to other methods of self-regulation such as progressive deep relaxation (shown to regulate heart rate), meditation, visualization, and imagery.

*Practitioners*—Biofeedback is now used in many medical clinics and psychological therapy centers.

*Conditions or illnesses best suited for*—Biofeedback training has proven especially effective for pain relief, stress reduction, and the management of headache and asthma.

## Chiropractic Medicine

Chiropractic means "done by the hand." Chiropractic practitioners believe many illnesses start when the vertebrae of the spinal column slip out of place and pinch nerves, cutting off the body's vital energy flow. To free blocked energy and balance the functions of the body, Chiropractic practitioners realign the spinal vertebrae by hand. Chiropractic is frequently used for neck, shoulder, arm, and back pain, slipped disks, other musculoskeletal pains, and headaches. Chiropractors also advise on nutrition, exercise, and rest and may employ other alternative therapies such as massage, acupressure, or yoga. The number of chiropractors in practice make this therapy one of the most widely recognized alternative medicine professions in the world.

*Usefulness*—Chiropractic medicine takes a holistic view of health, but the primary focus is the condition of the spinal column and nerves, along with the nervous system that extends through the body. Chiropractic is especially effective in treating back disorders. Severe back pain is one of the most widespread forms of suffering, with some eight out of ten Americans experiencing back pain before reaching fifty. It is also a treatment of choice for joint injuries, sprains, and arthritis.

*Research*—A study in the *British Medical Journal* titled "Low Back Pain of Mechanical Origin: Randomised Comparison of Chiropractic and Hospital Outpatient Treatment" states the Medical Research Council of Britain found chiropractic treatment more effective for low back pain than hospital outpatient care. The Rand Corporation Study published a study entitled "The Appropriateness of Spinal Manipulation for Low Back Pain: Indications and Ratings by a Multidisciplinary Expert Panel."

*Practitioners*—There are tens of thousands of licensed Doctors of Chiropractic, D.C., in every city and locality. Just look in the yellow pages.

*Conditions or illnesses best suited for*—Problems of the nervous and muscular system caused by pinched nerve trunks and misaligned vertebrae.

## Faith Healing

People have sought to heal the body through faith alone since ancient times. The use of faith healing and the touch of hands on the sick person was practiced by priests in the ancient temples of healing in Egypt. The practice of seeking healing from a higher source continues worldwide up to the present day. The early history of Christianity is replete with accounts of spiritual healing. In the *New Testament,* the "Book of James" says, "If anyone is sick, let them call for the elders of the church, and they shall anoint them with olive oil, and the prayer of faith will raise up the sick person." In the 103RD Psalm of David, it is written, "Praise the Lord, O my soul, and forget not all his benefits. He forgives all my sins and heals all my diseases."

Belief in the power of faith to effect physical healing is common to many religions. Although many people mistakenly believe that faith healing requires a faith healer to do the healing or to be its conduit, this is not true. Studies show the potential to administer faith healing, both to others and to one's self, is present in everyone. On the mind/body level, belief in the healing power of prayer, as well as the peace and well-being it brings, may create a positive physiological state that promotes well-being and strengthens the immune system.

*Usefulness*—In dozens of studies, patients who pray and are prayed for have recuperated faster than other patients.

*Research*—An experiment in the effect of prayer on healing at the Arthritis/Pain Treatment Center in Clearwater, Florida found that the degree of improvement in rheumatoid arthritis, was so strong it could be readily observed and measured. All the patients in the study were given standard medical care for their rheumatoid arthritis. A minister prayed for relief of the symptoms of one patient group being treated. Another group of patients received the same medical treatment but no prayers. The center's clinical staff examined the patients immediately after the experiment, a month later, then at three, six, and twelve month intervals and found the short term results of the study encouraging. After only four prayer sessions, one male patient, who started the experiment with forty-nine tender joints, was found to have only eight tender joints. When he was re-examined six months later, his arthritis improved so much, he no longer required medication for the pain. Not all patients have such spectacular results.

*Practitioners*—Prayer for the sick and healing by faith are practiced worldwide by those of all religious faiths.

*Comparisons*—The creation of a positive emotional attitude is similar to the mind/body medicines of visualization and imagery.

*Conditions or illnesses best suited for*—Every form of known illness has been the subject of intercessory prayer.

## Folk Medicine

Contemporary folk medicine is today's version of a system by which both man and animals have cured themselves for a millennia. Rural folk discovered the curative power of plants by observing how livestock reacted after eating them. They applied this knowledge and devised what came to be known as natural home remedies. This knowledge, refined by scientific knowledge, continues to keep people healthy.

The ideal of folk medicine is to condition the body in its entirety so disease will not attack it. This ideal is even more important today, when we realize the importance of our miraculous immune system protecting us from every threat from colds to cancer. One key notion in folk medicine is people should not abandon their ancestral or ethnic diet when making healthy food choices. For example, if you are Nordic or Northern European, your ancestors ate about ten times as much fish as they did red meat. You might want to give that pattern a try, to see if it provides any useful health benefits.

Folk medicine is still sworn by in areas like Vermont, where many natives use apple cider vinegar to maintain robust health in farmers and their dairy herds. This old folk remedy has recently been validated through modern research which shows the soils in Vermont are low in the essential mineral potassium, while apple cider vinegar is very rich in it. Apple cider vinegar can also help restore acid/alkaline imbalances. "The pain of paranasal sinusitis is associated with an alkaline-urine reaction," writes Dr. D.C. Jarvis, a graduate of the University of Vermont School of Medicine, and a fifth-generation Vermonter. He has found value in incorporating folk medicine and Western medicine in his practice. "As a rule, one can shift the reaction to acid, relieving the pain, by taking one tablespoon of apple cider vinegar in a glass of water each hour for seven doses."

Dr. Jarvis reports that two teaspoonfuls of apple cider vinegar, taken in a glass of pure water before eating, can provide additional protection to the digestive tract when the food is not of the best quality. Dr. Jarvis says many folk traditions consider honey to be a magnet for excess water in the body. Taken at mealtime, it is believed to draw excess fluid from the blood, lower blood pressure, and alleviate unhealthy tension in the nervous system.

Another benefit of folk medicine is its reliance on common sense solutions to promoting health with natural, inexpensive, and widely available plants. It is a system that still concentrates on the three Rs—resistance, repair, and recovery. Today's updated version is receiving scientific as well as popular validation. For example, garlic was known to the ancient Egyptians, who fed it to pyramid builders and soldiers as a means of fortifying the body and building strength. On long voyages, the intrepid Vikings and Phoenicians took along ample supplies of garlic cloves. Garlic, long a pillar of the healthy Mediterranean diet, is proven to be a blood thinner and natural antibiotic.

One alternative healing tradition that combines the scientific approach with folk medicine is naturopathy. Naturopathic Doctors (N.D.), who are graduates of accredited colleges of naturopathy, and are licensed to practice in some states and provinces, are modern keepers of folk medicine. There are also books on folk medicine and natural home remedies that can guide you further.

*Usefulness*—The ingredients for many of today's folk remedies are safe, inexpensive, and easily obtained. The overriding ideal of folk medicine is to keep the body healthy so disease will not attack it. It is a system both natural and preventive, something to be used every day for the maintenance and restoration of good health.

*Research*—Folk remedies have been tested in the clinical practice of physicians like D.C. Jarvis, M.D., and have been evaluated and taught in colleges of naturopathy. *Folk Medicine,* Galahad Books, 1996.

*Practitioners*—Folk medicine is integrated into the practice of a number of health professionals, including physicians, nurses, and naturopaths. It is well-suited for self care with proper guidance and instructions.

*Comparisons*—Folk medicine can be compared to other natural systems of healing, including naturopathy, herbal medicine, aromatherapy, traditional Chinese medicine, and Ayurvedic medicine.

*Conditions or illnesses best suited for*—Folk remedies are best for maintaining a strong immune system to prevent disease. When restoration is necessary, they provide a safe and inexpensive alternative, one that can work in a complementary way with conventional medicine.

## Food Therapy

The idea of food as medicine is not new. Hippocrates taught the concept back in the fifth century B.C. What is new is the breakthrough scientific research that has revealed the existence of heretofore unknown components of foods, components that are now known to have a powerful effect on getting well and staying well. It is a breakthrough in our understanding of health that many have compared to the discovery of germs and the role it played in our understanding of disease.

Prior to 1900, when America was a place of small farms with the whole foods of fresh produce and whole grains, the devastating diseases of heart trouble and cancer were rare or unknown. The first heart attack was described in 1908 in the *Journal of the American Medical Association.* Heart diseases are now our number one killers. The change from the nineteeenth century's low fat, high fiber, vegetable-based foods to today's high fat, low fiber, meat-centered foods is thought to be at the root of these diseases.

Found in all plants, phytochemicals are natural healing compounds thought to strengthen the plant's health and its long-term survival against pests and disease. But phytochemicals aren't just good for the plant's health, they're good for yours too. Even in small dosages, phytochemicals have been shown to be helpful protecting the body against a number of different cancers, especially those in the linings of organs such as the stomach, colon, rectum, larynx, lungs, pancreas, cervix, and bladder. Some plants especially rich in phytochemicals are:

- *Beans*—Be they kidney, pinto, or black, beans supply soluble fiber, which forms a gel in the intestines that prevents saturated fats from being absorbed into the body. So, if you must have that steak, or any other item rich in saturated fats, order some beans along with it. Maybe those chuck wagon cooks of the Old West, who were always being joshed for serving beans morning, noon, and night, knew what they were doing after all. Beans are also an excellent source of protein and B vitamins, along with other phytonutrients.

- *Citrus fruits*—Their rind contains bioflavonoids that prevent cancer-causing hormones from attaching to cells.

- *Garlic*—Contains the phytonutrients allicin and diallyl disulfide, which reduce blood pressure, help prevent blood clots, and reduce the less desirable LDL cholesterol in the blood.

- *Olive oil*—Studies have determined that olive oil should be used in place of butter or margarine. Olive oil has emerged as a first choice among food oils. High in monounsaturated fats, which lower cholesterol in the blood, it has a long history of proven health benefits as a staple of the Italian diet.

- *Onions*—Long reputed by folk medicine for its health-giving qualities, the onion was thought to be helpful in allergy attacks. Research has identified quercetin, an anti-inflammatory which is chemically similar to antihistamines, as the primary phytonutrient in onions. Quercetin isn't affected by heat, so you can eat onions raw or cooked.

- *Pineapple and green peppers*—Contain phytonutrients that prevent the formation of cancer cells.

- *Shiitake mushrooms*—The active phytochemical in the mushrooms is lentinan, which enhances the immune system by increasing the production of disease-fighting, white blood cells.

- *Strawberries*—Have the highest source of antioxidants in the fruit group. These phytochemicals are a prime preventive against free radical damage, which causes atherosclerosis, cancer, and other serious health problems.

- *Tomato sauce*—Contains lycopene, another antioxidant. A study of European men showed diets high in products containing tomatoes and tomato sauce, were 50 percent less likely to suffer a stroke or heart attack. Men whose diets were high in lycopene were also found to be at lower risk for prostate problems. While raw tomatoes are excellent health foods, cooking them releases five times more lycopene on average.

As always, food therapy recommends whole foods when practical. Whole grains with the bran in them, for instance, are better than taking the bran by itself as a supplement. Whole foods are designed with an intelligence far beyond our own.

Another key principle of food as therapy is to eat lots of vegetables. They are filled with many diverse and complex nutrients, ranging from vitamins and minerals to phytochemicals. Vegetables are diffuse foods, they're filled with water, so you need a lot of them. Have big salads for lunch. If you're concerned about your weight, don't be, most people who eat large amounts of fruits and vegetables lose weight.

*Cancer Preventive Foods*

Here are a few of the most highly recommended:

- *Soybean products*—Shown to contain genistein, which may help prevent breast cancer, and Indol-3-carbinol, which reduces levels of specific estrogen compounds in the bloodstream. Many alternative health care practitioners recommended that you add soy products to your meals two or more times a week.

- *Cabbage*—Another source of Indol-3-carbinol, as well as some other anticancer compounds.

- *Black tea*—Contains polyphenols, which help reduce the risk of cancer.

- *Green tea*—An effective antioxidant.

- *Grapes*—Contain resveratrol, a cancer inhibitor that may cause precancerous cells to return to normal. Researchers recommend eating whole grapes, in addition to red wine or grape juice, to get the entire spectrum of resveratrol's beneficial effects.

*Usefulness*—Food therapy is useful for maintaining health as well as preventing disease.

*Research*—Heart disease, cancer, stroke, and diabetes, four of the leading causes of death in America, have been linked to diet. According to Basil Rifkind, M.D., of the National Heart, Lung, and Blood Institute in Bethesda, Maryland, diet is the single largest contributor to the number one cause of death in the U.S.—heart disease.

A 1996 study reported that women who drank two or more cups of black tea a day had up to a 60 percent reduced cancer risk. Tea contains polyphenols, which inhibit the formation of carcinogens. Ronald Watson, Ph.D., research professor and immunology specialist at the University of Arizona College of Medicine, reports that a healthy diet becomes more important as you grow older. Immunity tends to weaken as time passes, placing you at greater risk for infection and cancer.

*Practitioners*—Food therapy is practiced by nutritional specialists, nutritional consultants, alternative health care providers, and conventional physicians and health care providers. With sound information and guidance, it is suitable for self care.

*Comparisons*—Food therapy can be compared to vitamin and mineral therapy. The difference is that with food therapy the micronutrients are obtained by consuming the macronutrients as foods that contain the vitamins, minerals, and other nutrients. Both systems seek to prevent health problems and enhance life by providing the body with the necessary nutrients.

*Conditions or illnesses best suited for*—Food therapy is best for building up the body's vitality and the immune system's resistant powers. The risk of diseases linked to diet, including cancer and heart disease, can be almost entirely eliminated.

## Herbs and Herbal Medicine

Herbal medicine has been around for four thousand years. Herbs are described in ancient Egyptian papyrus, and were used by the Greek, Roman, and Islamic peoples. Herbs are a mainstay of the healing systems in India, Tibet, and China. Every culture in the world has venerated these products of the earth's natural pharmacy for their tonic and healing properties.

Health food stores now stock an impressive variety of herbal products, along with books, guides, and advice on how to use them. Herbs are now being prescribed and recommended by both Western physicians and alternative health care providers. The recommendations of herbalist James A. Duke for a variety of conditions are listed in the chart on the chart on the following page.

Some popular herbs at your health food store include:

### HERBAL REMEDIES

| Condition | Herbal Remedy | Replace Drug Store Remedy |
|---|---|---|
| Allergies | Garlic, stinging nettle, ginkgo | Synthetic antihistamines |
| Body odor, perspiration | Coriander, sage | Deodorants |
| Colds | Echinacea, ginger, lemon balm, garlic | Decongestants |
| Cuts & scrapes | Tea tree oil, calendula, plantain (all external) | Topical antibiotic |
| Earache | Echinacea, garlic, mullein | Antibiotics |
| Flu | Echinacea, elderberry | Acetaminophen |
| Headache | Peppermint (external), feverfew, willow | Aspirin |
| Heartburn | Angelica, chamomile, peppermint | Antacids |
| Indigestion | Chamomile, ginger, peppermint | Antacids |
| Low back pain | Cayenne (external), thyme | Analgesics |
| Motion sickness | Ginger | Pills |
| Stress | Kava kava, valerian | Tranquilizers |

- *St. John's wort*—Used as a mood lifter and antidepressant.

- *Ginkgo*—Used by many people as a brain tonic, to sharpen mental performance and memory.

- *Garlic*—An old friend to most cooks, is winning friends as a natural medicine with antibiotic, antiviral, and antifungal properties. Garlic is considered a natural preventive against colds and flu, and a winner for your heart. It is recommended for people with elevated lipid (liquid fat) levels in their blood.

- *Hawthorn berries*—A favorite heart tonic in natural medicine, with cardiotonic and hypotensive properties.

- *Milk thistle*—Research shows the milk thistle can be an important agent in reversing toxic liver damage, and protecting the liver from other toxins.

- *Saw palmetto*—Known to be an effective treatment for the enlargement of the prostate gland; also thought to strengthen the reproductive system.

*Usefulness*—Herbal remedies are used as preventive medicine and alleviating specific illnesses. Herbal medicine constitutes a whole natural pharmacy of its own. Many of the drugs used in Western medicine were originally derived from similar plant sources.

*Research*—An abundance of scientific research has demonstrated the effectiveness of herbs and herbal medicine. It is estimated that over one thousand research projects have been devoted to garlic alone, for example, HerbalGram's "Anticancer Effects of Garlic— More Proof." Another example of research on garlic was published in the *British Journal of Clinical Pharmacology*, entitled "Garlic, Onions, and Cardiovascular Risk Factors."

In Germany, where St. John's wort is frequently prescribed by doctors as an antidepressant, a study was done on "Antidepressant Effect of a Hypericum Extract Standardized to an Active Hypericine Complex. Biochemical and Clinical Studies."

*Comparisons*—Herbal medicine can be compared to aromatherapy, traditional Chinese medicine, and Ayurvedic medicine, all of whom use plants and herbs in their remedies.

*Conditions or illnesses best suited for*—A wide range of health needs that are suitable to self care.

## Homeopathy

Homeopathy, which literally means "treatment by the same," was developed by the German doctor and chemist Samuel

Hahnemann (1755–1843). Homeopathy is based on the principle that a drug taken in small amounts will cure the disease symptoms it causes in large amounts. Hahnemann found that chinchona, whose active component is quinine, a cure for malaria, gave him the symptoms of malaria, even though he did not have the disease. He had rediscovered the principle of "like can cure like," a natural approach to health whose value he proved in a series of experiments.

Homeopathy links health to temperament and divides people into constitutional types according to physical and emotional characteristics. Homeopathic remedies range from common foods like honey, to toxic substances like snake venom. However, homeopathic remedies are diluted so greatly before use there is little danger even from the most seemingly toxic of substances in the homeopathic pharmacopoeia. This gives the practice its reputation as a gentle approach to healing.

Homeopathy is a large and well-organized system of medicine. There are medical schools and hospitals for the training of homeopathic physicians, and many professionally trained homeopaths in North America and the United Kingdom have physician degrees. Homeopathic remedies are prescribed by some conventional physicians for a number of problems. Homeopathic remedies are also available in health food stores. For more detail, see the many books on the subject, such as *The Complete Guide to Homeopathy*, by Dr. Andrew Lockie and Dr. Nicola Geddes.

*Usefulness*—Homeopathic physicians report that this therapy has been effective in the reversal of arthritis, allergies, bronchial asthma, diabetes, dermatologic conditions, and some emotional and mental disorders.

*Research*—A study in the *British Medical Journal* titled "Clinical Trials of Homeopathy" detailed over one hundred clinical studies performed between 1966 and 1990. Eighty-one of the studies indicated that homeopathic remedies benefited many health problems, including sprained ankles, digestive disorders, respiratory infections, and headaches.

The *British Journal of Clinical Pharmacology* published the results of a study on "A Controlled Evaluation of a Homeopathic Preparation for the Treatment of Influenza-like Symptoms." In two groups of patients, one taking a homeopathic preparation and one taking a placebo, twice as many patients in the group taking the homeopathic preparation were cured within forty-eight hours, compared to the group who took a placebo.

*Comparisons*—In the use of very dilute substances to achieve therapeutic results, homeopathy can be compared to the Bach flower remedies, and to aromatherapy.

*Conditions or illnesses best suited for*—Homeopathic physicians report this therapy is especially effective in the prevention and treatment of colds and flu, and in treating chronic illnesses.

## Hydrotherapy

Hydrotherapy is the use of water to promote wellness and healing. It is another ancient art that has been refined into a modern science. Today it is frequently used by naturopathic doctors, and other alternative therapists. In Europe, especially Germany, hydrotherapy is very much in favor. The health benefits of warm, healing springs, and cold, bracing ones have been celebrated throughout history and around the world. It is the basis of the therapeutic regimes at many spas, which not so coincidentally are usually parked next to a natural spring. Anyone who has ever taken a hot bath or a cold shower knows that water and water temperature can have an extraordinary effect on the body and nervous system.

"To understand how something as simple as the application of water could profoundly affect the body, we must review the mechanisms of heat regulation," writes Dr. Ross Trattler, a naturopathic physician, "since it is by these basic bodily responses that hydrotherapy is able to produce its reactions." He goes on to say, "Nervous reflexes produced by heating the skin inhibit these centers and vasodilation results. This dilation of the blood vessels occurs not only in and about the heated area, but also in other areas reflexly related. It is in this distant reflex response that most of the beneficial results of the superficial application of heat occur for the treatment of internal disorders. The effects of cold on the body are controlled primarily by the nervous system. Heat loss is reduced by superficial vasoconstriction of blood vessels. As a general rule, the shorter the application and the more extreme the temperature, the more purely excitant will be the effect of hot or cold."

Because of individual differences in people, and the strain any great temperature change puts on the body, careful consideration must be given to the state of your health when beginning hydrotherapy. Treatments should be conducted under the supervision of a qualified therapist or after consulting your own health practitioner.

Hydrotherapy methods include:

- *Whirlpool*—Used in physiotherapy as well, it is an effective way to rehabilitate weakened, diseased, or injured muscles. The whirlpool is also beneficial to those recovering from stroke and certain forms of paralysis.

- *Hyperthermia*—Heat can be applied in a hot tub, deep hot bath (103 to 104 degrees Fahrenheit), or a steam room. Heat acts as a powerful dilator of blood vessels, and should be administered carefully under proper supervision.

- *Ice packs*—Ideal for treating injuries, acute muscle strain or spasm, inflamed joints or tendonitis. In most cases, it is advised to apply the pack twenty minutes of every hour for the first one or two days after an injury.

- *Sitz baths*—In a sitz bath you sit with water up to your navel, usually hot water, for a minimum of fifteen minutes. Sitz baths are recommended for conditions such as hemorrhoids, fissures, prostatitis, vaginal irritation, and menstrual cramps.

*Usefulness*—Hydrotherapy is considered a very safe and useful form of therapy, and is used by both alternative and conventional medical practitioners.

*Research*—A study in the *British Journal of Radiology* reported their laboratory research showed HIV (human immunodeficiency virus) was sensitive to temperature and displayed greater inactivation per unit of time at progressively higher temperatures above the normal body temperature of 98.6 degrees Fahrenheit. Another publication, *The Body/Mind Purification Program,* described how the hydrotherapy methods of alternating between hot and cold water during a treatment were beneficial in improving blood circulation, stimulating certain organs, and alleviating congestion.

*Practitioners*—Hydrotherapy is used by naturopaths and many branches of conventional and alternative medicine. Medical experts consider it a safe therapy when normal cautions of heat and duration are observed. It is a therapy suitable for home use and self care.

*Comparisons*—Hydrotherapy is used by physiotherapists and in rehabilitation medicine.

*Conditions or illnesses best suited for*—Whirlpool: Rehabilitating injured, weakened, or diseased muscles. Ice packs: Inflamed joints, tendonitis, acute muscle strain or spasm. Hot water: dilating blood vessels.

## Hypnotherapy

Hypnosis is a method of therapy used to treat diverse conditions from insomnia, to addiction to tobacco, to bed-wetting. In the opinion of some experts, it is a way for the client to take greater control of their own health. The hypnotherapist is seen as a facilitator in the process.

Research scientists now recognize that body functions controlled by the autonomic system, such as blood circulation, can be affected by the mind and emotions. Hypnosis, correctly applied, may allow access to the controls that control emotions. In the case of insomnia, a usual method is to teach the client self hypnosis slowly, allowing them to relax and then sleep. In the case of enuresis, or bed-wetting, mild forms of positive suggestions are used, telling the subject when they have a need they will awaken by themselves, take care of the need by themselves, and return to their nice, dry bed. They are told that when they awaken in a dry bed they will feel very happy. Only suggestions for positive behavior are made.

Health care providers, such as physicians, psychologists, and dentists, may also provide hypnosis therapy. Their extensive knowledge of the workings of the mind and body are of great value in the application of hypnotherapy. Hypnotherapy was approved as a valid medical treatment by the British Medical Association in 1955. It was approved by the American Medical Association in 1958.

*Usefulness*—Hypnotherapy is a useful non-drug method for changing behaviors in cases of cigarette smoking, alcohol abuse, and overeating. It is also used medically for pain relief, and for emotional and psychological therapy. The World Health Organization advises that hypnosis should not be used on people with antisocial personality disorders, organic psychiatric illness, or psychosis.

*Research*—In "Hypnotherapy for Chronic Pain," the *Kansas Medicine* journal reported that hypnotherapy had been used to control pain in chronic ailments such as osteoarthritis, rheumatoid arthritis, headaches, menstrual pain, sciatica, tennis elbow, and whiplash.

An article in *The American Surgeon* described "The Use of Hypnotic Anesthesia for Major Surgical Procedure." Hypnotherapy was substituted for conventional anesthetics in abdominal surgery, the treatment of serious burns, and other major surgical procedures.

*Practitioners*—Hypnotherapists, psychologists, physicians.

*Conditions or illnesses best suited for*—Treating addictions to tobacco, alcohol, and other substances, and for cases of overeating. Useful in stress management and in emotional and psychological therapy. Effective in pain relief.

## Juice Therapy

Drinking the fresh juices of vegetables and fruits has long been considered the very essence of health. In juice therapy, the emphasis is on fresh juices you prepare yourself and drink within thirty minutes of juicing, while they are still at their most nutritious.

One of the great benefits of raw juices is that they pass on plant energy that has been created by photosynthesis in sunlight, along with the minerals the plants have drawn from the earth, and the vitamins, enzymes, phytochemicals, and other nutrients the plant has produced. Thus, when you are drinking fresh juice, you are literally drinking in the life-giving energy of nature.

The juices of fresh vegetables and fruits has been proven to be the single richest and best source of vitamins, minerals, and health-giving enzymes. Juices are nutrient dense. Ideally, you might obtain the same number of nutrients from eating an ideal diet of whole foods—fruits, vegetables, and grains, along with their juice, pulp, and fiber. But such a diet is not practical for everyone. Fruits and vegetables are diffuse foods, filled with water, and you have to eat a lot of them to get the same amount of nutrients as in a glass of vegetable or fruit juice.

Fresh fruits and vegetables contain compounds that have profound protective effects on the body. That is why the National Research Council, the National Cancer Institute, the American Cancer Society, and other health committees worldwide urge you to eat them daily. Are you eating two servings of fruits and seven servings of vegetables every day? Is the ratio at which you eat these foods 60 percent raw and 40 percent cooked? It is the raw foods that contain the enzymes and other nutrients that are often destroyed in processing, storage, and cooking.

Authors Leslie and Susannah Kenton write that a vast quantity of evidence exists showing that the high-raw diet—a way of eating in which 75 percent of your foods are taken raw—cannot only reverse the bodily degeneration which accompanies long-term illness, but retard the rate at which you age, bring you seemingly boundless energy, and even make you feel better emotionally." However, studies show that most of us only eat one to three salads weekly. Experts say juice therapy is the only way most people can get enough fresh nutrients they need to be really fit, vital, and enjoy a longer life.

Physician Max Gerson, M.D., found when nothing else seemed to work, he put his cancer patients on a juice therapy regimen, and many of them regained their health. The late Max Bircher-Benner, M.D., who founded the Bircher-Benner clinic in Europe, hailed vegetable juice as the most therapeutic form of nutrition on earth. Proponents even credit juice therapy with healing thousands of sick people whose doctors had diagnosed their condition as terminal.

There are many books detailing specific juices and juice blends to cure specific illnesses in health food stores. One such remedy advises those plagued with insomnia to drink a blend of freshly juiced celery and lettuce leaves thirty minutes before bedtime as an aid to sleep.

*Usefulness*—Juice therapy is the most compact form in which to take in the fresh, raw nutrients your body needs to maintain health.

*Research*—In his book, *A Cancer Therapy: Results of Fifty Cases*, Max Gerson, M.D., reports on fifty patients, all of whom recovered from cancer through his treatments, which included juice therapy. The journal *Carcinogenesis* reported that onions and garlic oil inhibit tumor growth. (Onions and garlic are included in juicing recipes.) The British medical journal *Lancet* reported on the use of banana in non-ulcer dyspepsia.

Juice therapy can address vitamin supplementation through juice recipes known to be good sources of the vitamin. For example, a good source of vitamin E can be obtained by juicing three asparagus spears, four carrots, and one quarter cup of spinach.

*Practitioners*—Physicians, nutritionists, and other health counselors. Used by individuals for self care to promote vitality and longevity.

*Comparisons*—Juice therapy can be compared to food therapy and to vitamin and mineral therapy. It is a nutritional approach to healing in the area of nutritional medicine.

*Conditions or illnesses best suited for*—All illnesses resulting from nutritional deficiencies, or a body lacking in vital physical energy.

## Macrobiotics

Macrobiotics has been described as a philosophy that takes a wide or large (macro) view of life (biotics). The present practice of macrobiotics arose in Japan as a personal philosophy involving wholesome living and eating. Food is considered central to life, and the macrobiotic diet is selected with great care. The principles of yin and yang, the theory of opposites, is the guiding decision in determining foods for the diet. Cereal grains, for example, are considered an ideal food because they contain a balance of both yin and yang, and have become the staple of the macrobiotic diet comprising about half of every meal.

Benefits include a way of healthy eating that includes plenty of cereal fiber, fresh fruits and vegetables, very little red meat, and no processed or refined foods. Macrobiotics focuses on cooked foods, and can be applied to a vegetarian or non-vegetarian diet—but dairy products are prohibited. Though macrobiotics emphasizes grains, a good macrobiotic diet should also include a range of food products as nutritional experts advise avoiding going to extremes in choices of diets. A broadly based macrobiotic diet can be a healthy one.

Macrobiotics believes that illness cannot develop in a balanced body. Eating the wrong foods, thinking the wrong thoughts, missing sleep, or some other lifestyle problems throw this natural balance off. Macrobiotic practitioners diagnose whether too much yin or yang is present in the body, then redress the imbalance with increased amounts of food of the opposite polarity.

The concept of macrobiotics originated with an educator named Yukikazu Sakurazawa and a physician named Sagen Ishisuka (who later took on the pen name of George Oshawa). At one time, in the early 1900s, when much of the Japanese population was choosing a diet of refined foods, these two men found health by returning to a simple diet of brown rice, miso soup, sea vegetables, and other traditional Japanese foods. The two men went on to integrate other teachings—such as traditional Oriental medicine, holistic principles in modern science, and spiritual principles from Vedanta and original Christian and Jewish teachings— into macrobiotics.

A preeminent teacher in the movement is Michio Kushi who studied with George Oshawa at the Student World Government Association in Japan. Oshawa believed food was the key to health and health was the key to peace. He believed humanity could regain its physical and mental balance, and by doing so become more peaceful, if they would return to a traditional diet of whole, natural foods. After studies at Tokyo University and Columbia University, Kushi studied traditional and modern principles of diet and health, and began to teach macrobiotics as a way to world peace. In 1978 he founded the Kushi Institute for One Peaceful World.

Michio Kushi describes today's macrobiotics as "a unique synthesis of Eastern and Western influences. It is the way of life according to the largest possible view, the infinite order of the universe. The practice of macrobiotics involves the understanding and practical application of this order to our lifestyle, including the selection, preparation, and manner of eating our daily food, as well as the orientation of our consciousness. Macrobiotics does not offer a single diet for everyone, but a dietary principle that takes into account differing climactic and geographical considerations, varying ages, sexes, and levels of activity, and ever-changing personal needs."

Kushi teaches that macrobiotics is a cancer-prevention diet, and other proponents tout it as an excellent preventive of heart disease.

*Usefulness*—Macrobiotics offers the user the choice of a diet and a philosophy of life which may serve as a health-promoting alternative regimen for some people.

*Research*—An article in the journal *Cancer* entitled, "Diet and Breast Cancer Causation and Therapy" suggests breast cancer patients on high fat diets have poorer survival times than those on low fat diets. The article concludes, "We are surprised that most physicians pay so little attention to the likelihood that metabolic overloads in terms of nutritional intake could have a deleterious effect, aside from the obvious obesity, on many bodily functions. Therefore, nutritional adjustments are very likely to be an effective pharmacologic intervention, particularly when used early in the disease process; in fact, 'we are what we eat.'"

A study by Barry R. Goldin of the New England Medical Center Hospital in Boston compared the excretion of estrogens in healthy pre- and post-menopausal macrobiotic and omnivorous women. They found that vegetarian (macrobiotic) women excrete two to three times more estrogens in feces than do those who eat meat, and that women who eat meat have about 50 percent higher plasma levels of estrogen products than do vegetarians. "[The] data suggest that in vegetarians a greater amount of the biliary estrogens escape reabsorption (in the intestines) and are excreted with the feces. The differences in estrogen metabolism may explain the lower incidence of breast cancer in vegetarian women."

In another study, published in the journal *Nutrition and Cancer*, Takeshi Hirayama at the National Cancer Center Research Institute in Japan reported that daily intake of soybean paste (miso) soup correlated with dramatically reduced gastric cancer rates in a large-scale study of over 260,000 Japanese men and women. The researchers noted that the benefits could result from compounds such as protease inhibitors or other nutritious factors in the soybean paste. They might also come from beneficial foods that often are eaten with soybean soup, such as green and yellow vegetables.

*Practitioners*—Health counselors, members of the macrobiotic community, other users for self care.

*Comparisons*—The macrobiotic diet is, to a large degree, derived from the traditional Japanese diet.

*Conditions or illnesses best suited for*—Macrobiotics benefit any condition that can be improved by an extremely healthy, primarily vegetarian, high complex carbohydrate, low fat diet.

## Massage and Other Forms of Bodywork

Massage and bodywork seek to heal the body by releasing blocked energy, much like acupuncture, acupressure, and chiropractic. The Touch Research Institute of Miami University has demonstrated the benefits of massage for people in a spectrum of illnesses, including asthma, back pain, chronic fatigue syndrome, cystic fibrosis, diabetes, fibromyalgia, immune deficiency disorders, atherosclerosis, rheumatoid arthritis, skin disorders, addictions, carpal tunnel syndrome, burns, cancer, spinal cord injuries, and high blood pressure. The benefits of massage come from improved sleep, relief from depression, anxiety, and fatigue, reduced output of stress hormones, and greater vigor.

Bodywork incorporates a host of therapies that manipulate the body in different ways to promote health, among them Rolfing, the Alexander Technique, and Trager work. The Office of Alternative Medicine, a department of the National Institutes of Health, estimates that 20 million Americans have tried bodywork since the 1970s, many for specific medical complaints. Others show that massage and other bodywork therapies confer real health benefits. Many hospitals are now using massage as an adjunct to other therapies. In some ways the rising tide of bodywork therapies marks a return to days when massage was taught to doctors in medical school, and was practiced as an important means of treatment.

*"The physician must be experienced in many things, but assuredly also in rubbing... For rubbing can bind a joint which is too loose and loosen a joint that is too hard."*
—*Hippocrates*

### Reflexology

Reflexology is based on the theory that there are important energy meridians that end at specific points in the feet and hands and link to specific body organs and systems. Reflexology, sometimes called Zone Therapy, teaches that the body is divided into ten energy zones, running from the top of the head to the toes. Five energy zones are on the left side of the body, and five are on the right. By massaging shiatsu meridian points within a zone, the therapist can affect the energy in another part of the same zone, releasing the flow of energy to any organs or systems that are blocked off.

Benefits of reflexology are indicated as relaxation and relief from stress and an overall increase in energy. Reflexology is often recommended for stress related disorders, such as headaches, backaches, chronic indigestion, and high blood pressure. Many other physical ailments are said to be aided by the therapy.

### Rolfing

Also known as structural integration, Rolfing was developed by Ida Rolf, Ph.D. Rolf believed that humans function in improved ways when the segments of their body—feet, legs, pelvis, torso, head—are correctly aligned. When the body's physical structure is out of alignment, disease sets in. Rolf wrote that, "One individual may experience his losing fight with gravity as a sharp pain in the back, another as the unflattering contour of his body, another as a constant fatigue, and yet another as an unrelenting threatening environment. Those over forty may call it old age; yet all these signals may be pointing to a single problem so prominent in their own structures that it has been ignored: they are off-balance; they are all at war with gravity."

In Rolfing, structural integration is intended to restore the body to optimum alignment and balance. Structural integration can be described as an extremely deep massage that stretches connective tissue, promoting the release of lactic acid. Rolfing works on the fascia, the membrane sheaths covering the muscles.

Rolfing is well-suited to relieve chronic, rather than acute pain. Benefits are relief from aches and pains resulting from poor posture, a sense of general well-being, greater ease and freedom in body movement, and improved energy. "For it is not structure alone," Rolf has said, "but the integration of structure that is the key. We seek to create a whole that is greater than the sum of its parts. We are searching for a method to foster the emergence of a man who can enjoy a human use of his human being."

*Research*—The journal *Human Behavior* reports that after rolfing posture was improved and more easily maintained, body movements were more energetic, smoother, and less constrained.

*Shiatsu*

The word comes from a Japanese word that literally means "finger pressure." It is a massage technique that is centered on pressure applied to the body by the fingers and palms of the hands, and sometimes with elbows, knees, and feet. Shiatsu can be thought of as a combination of acupressure and massage. Like reflexology, shiatsu creates its health benefit by applying pressure to twelve meridians on the body which channel physical, spiritual, and emotional energy. Each meridian travels partly through the body, connecting with various organs, and partly over the surface of the

The Meridian System: Front and Back Views

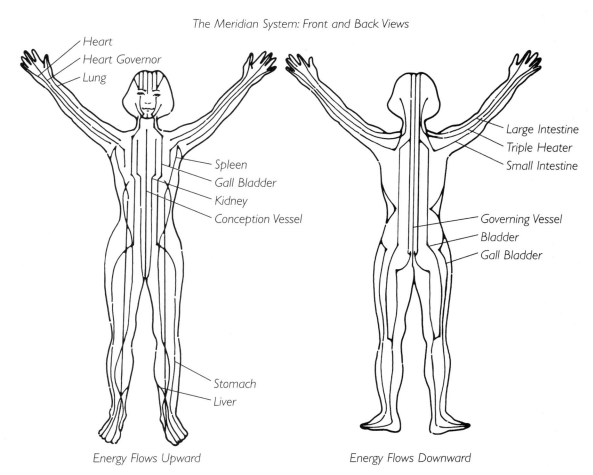

Energy Flows Upward

Energy Flows Downward

body. Each of the body's organs and systems are thought to be linked to a specific meridian and to suffer ill health when the energy flow along that meridian is blocked. By putting pressure on key points along these meridians, the shiatsu practitioner seeks to restore the vital flow of life force, enabling the body to heal itself. Benefits of shiatsu treatment are a general sense of well-being and help with chronic ailments, such as digestive problems. Research suggests that shiatsu also stimulates the release of endorphins, which are pain killers naturally found in the body.

The foundation of shiatsu dates back over two thousand years to *The Yellow Emperor's Classic of Internal Medicine,* which contains information on the cure of many different illnesses that can be remedied by changes in life style, diet, and with treatment by acupressure and massage. The Chinese form of massage was brought to Japan, where it was called *anma.* In modern times, new influences on *anma,* both from Eastern and Western medicine, have shaped it into the theory now known as shiatsu.

Shiatsu, like yoga, also includes stretching exercises that a person can do alone to stimulate the free flow of energy through the meridians and promote continued physical well-being.

*Usefulness*—Shiatsu benefits problems such as back pain, headaches, migraines, other aches, pains, or chronic tension in the body, insomnia, irregularities of menstrual cycles or painful periods, low libido or vitality, and prevalent negative moods like depression, anxiety, or worry.

*Research*—Research indicates that shiatsu treatments trigger the release of endorphins, and other natural pain killers in the body.

*Practitioners*—Most large cities have shiatsu practitioners who can be found in the yellow pages or through local workshops and health food stores.

*Comparisons*—Shiatsu can be compared to acupuncture.

*Conditions or illnesses best suited for*—Most people experience a feeling of relaxation and rejuvenation after a treatment by shiatsu. Clients report feeling more relaxed, sleeping better, feeling lighter and more alive, becoming more flexible by releasing areas of tension. Problems like backache, headache, or tired eyes disappear along with a feeling that a weight has been lifted from their shoulders.

### Sports Massage

Medicine has played an increasing role in helping athletes train to peak condition and recovery from any damage or strains incurred while playing. Sports massage focuses on areas of the body used in, or injuries through, physical exercise.

### Swedish Massage

The technique derives its name from the nationality of its founder, Per Heinrik Ling, a Swede who developed the therapy in the early 1800s. Practitioners stretch contracted muscles, relieving neck and lower back pains caused by tension and massage the muscles in long strokes that always move in the direction of the heart. This is thought to release toxins clogging the flow of lymph and blood. Ling's techniques have become the foundation of bodywork. The main objective of Swedish massage is to induce general relaxation while improving circulation and range of motion. Benefits include relief of overworked muscles and chronic muscle pain, as well as help with recovery from sciatica, sprains, and fractures.

### Trager Work

The Trager approach to bodywork uses gentle shaking, rocking, and bouncing motions to release tension and overcome rigidity and free the body so it can move through its full range of motion. Mental gymnastics, dancelike movements, and exercises are also used to enhance freedom of movement and greater awareness of how the body moves.

The purpose of the Trager approach is to help the patient recognize and release habitual patterns of tension that are present in posture and movement. Tension often leads to back, neck, and shoulder pain and loss of mobility in these areas and Trager work has provided relief for all these conditions. The *Trager Journal* reported that another objective in Trager approach is the use of movement in joints and muscles to achieve positive emotional and physical states in the client. These feelings were thought to benefit the central nervous system and initiate positive physical changes in the body's state of well-being.

The Trager system was developed by Milton Trager, who earned an M.D. degree at age forty-seven, and went on to combine his personal method of movement, education, and bodywork with his medical practice. Trager work has been used successfully to aid people with injuries or diseases of the neuromuscular system, from sprains and lower back pain, to multiple sclerosis, polio, Parkinson's disease, and post-stroke trauma. It has also been effective in treating asthma, emphysema, migraine headaches, and other conditions. It is part of the system prescribed for the treatment of sports-related injuries at the Elite Athlete Program in Austin, Texas.

Of his approach to bodywork, which some have called meditation in motion, Dr. Trager had this to say, "Many times after a real good session with a patient, I get so moved by their face that I must take them by the hand, take them to a mirror, and say 'I want you to meet this person.' Sometimes they say, 'I haven't seen her in twenty-five years.' What I feel is that this is actually the soul of the individual uncovered." Some clients even report Trager work has brought them a sense of relaxation, mental clarity, and creativity, and an experience of peace that lies beyond relaxation.

### Trigger Point Therapy

This is a form of bodywork that involves pressure applied directly to specific locations where there is irritation or pain in the muscles. Trigger points are tender areas, usually found in tight bands of muscle, that radiate pain to other areas of the body. Trigger points can result from a number of causes, including direct trauma to the body, exposure to cold, overloading, or overuse. While it shares some similarities to shiatsu and acupressure, Trigger Point therapy uses the anatomy of the body as described in conventional medicine. A variation of this technique is also known as Bonnie Prudden myotherapy, after the developer of that therapy, fitness authority Bonnie Prudden.

Janet Travell, M.D., White House physician to Presidents Kennedy and Johnson, was a developer and practitioner of Trigger Point therapy, and used it successfully to treat John F. Kennedy's chronic pain.

Conditions that have been treated with Trigger Point therapy include muscle lower back pain, TMJ, tennis elbow, and whiplash.

*Research*—In her book, *Pain Erasure,* Bonnie Prudden reported that 90 percent of muscle-related pain could be relieved by a simple finger pressure of five to seven seconds, applied to trigger points. Research was carried out in connection with Desmond Tivy, M.D., who had been active in the therapy known as trigger point injection, a technique developed by Janet Travell, M.D.

## Meditation

"Meditation is simply focusing your awareness on something," writes Dean Ornish, M.D., in *Stress, Diet, and Your Heart.* "It can be anything—your breathing, a part of your body, a sound, an activity." (For more detailed information on meditation, its benefits, and sample exercises see Chapter 5.)

Meditation has taken an important place in the modern healing arts and self care. It now plays an important part in many post-operative recovery and stress reduction programs. Western physicians prescribe it to those suffering from heart disease, cancer, asthma, and dozens of other illnesses.

Among the physicians and scientists who have established the health-giving benefits of meditation are:

Herbert Benson, M.D., a professor of medicine at Harvard Medical School, who has documented that regular meditation can reduce blood pressure significantly in those with hypertension, as well as decrease the frequency of irregular heartbeats (arrhythmias) in heart patients. He also found that alpha brain waves, which are present when people feel relaxed, increase in intensity and frequency during meditation, while muscular tension decreases measurably.

Dean Ornish, M.D. writes, "The physiological effects of profound relaxation produced by meditation are beneficial to people with coronary heart disease. In people who meditate, the oxygen consumption decreases 10 to 20 percent; this decrease begins during the first three minutes of meditation."

Andrew Weil, M.D. has written, "Researchers have documented immediate benefits in terms of lowered blood pressure, decreased heart and respiratory rate, increased blood flow, and other measurable signs of the relaxation response."

*Usefulness*—Research in the field of psychoneuroimmunology suggests meditation may be the single best remedy for stress and tensions, and the illnesses they cause. It also plays an important role in such techniques as visualization and imagery therapy.

*Research*—An article in the *Journal of Clinical Psychology* entitled "The Effects of Meditation and Relaxation Techniques on Trait Anxiety: A Meta-Analysis" concluded that meditation increased self-actualization and decreased anxiety. The *Journal of Transpersonal Psychology* published an article on "A Preliminary Study of Long Term Meditators: Goals, Effects, Religious Orientation, Cognitions" in which researcher Dean Shapiro, Ph.D. of the University of California, Irvine, reports that meditators who averaged four years of practicing the discipline of meditation highly rated the benefit of being able to control stress. Additional benefits include greater relaxation and control over negative thoughts.

In an article in the *Australian Family Physician*, psychiatrist Dr. Ainslie Meares, M.D. reported that nearly all the cancer patients in one study who participated in a minimum of twenty sessions of meditation experienced less anxiety, discomfort, depression, and pain. Benefits included a slowed growth of tumors and a 50 percent improvement in the quality of life.

In his *Full Catastrophe Living: Using the Wisdom of Your Body and Mind to Face Stress, Pain and Illness*, J. Kabat-Zinn, Ph.D. reported a study in which patients with chronic pain took part in an eight-week program of meditation. Kabat-Zinn wrote that 72 percent of the patients achieved at least a 33 percent reduction in their chronic pain, and 61 percent of the patients achieved at least 50 percent less pain.

*Conditions or illnesses best suited for*—Regulating high blood pressure, anxiety, and stress, strengthening the immune system in cancer patients, and normalizing brain rhythms in the treatment of drug and alcohol addiction.

## Naturopathy

Naturopathy is another medical philosophy which uses herbal medicines and other plant substances to release the body's inner vitality and aid the body in healing itself. It helps patients achieve wellness without drugs or surgery. Therapies used in naturopathic medicine include spinal manipulation, nutritional counseling, hydrotherapy, herbal medicine, aromatherapy, homeopathy, massage, and physiotherapy.

Hippocrates is considered the father of naturopathic medicine and his principles of healing are the foundation of naturopathy to this day. Hippocrates once said that only nature heals, meaning the body has a natural ability to heal itself. The methods he used included herbs, hydrotherapy, spinal manipulation, exercise, diet, and fasting.

Dr. Ross Trattler, a naturopathic physician, makes the following point, "The use of natural therapy does not of its own constitute naturopathy. Naturopathy involves the use of natural therapies according to certain established principles. This is where naturopathy as a science must be distinguished from folk medicine or any other natural therapy. While these techniques or tools may be employed by the naturopath, they must be used according to the basic principles of naturopathy for the end result to be naturopathic medicine."

In *The Philosophy of Natural Therapeutics,* Henry Lindlahr describes the philosophy of the naturopathic approach to medicine this way: "The natural therapeutic approach maintains that the constant effort of the body's life force is always in the direction of self-cleansing, self-repairing, and positive health. The philosophy maintains that even acute disease is a manifestation of the body's efforts in the direction of self cure. Disease, or downgraded health, may be eliminated only by removing from the system the real cause and by raising the body's general vitality so that its natural and inherent ability to sustain health is allowed to dominate. Natural therapeutic philosophy also maintains that chronic diseases are frequently the result of mistaken efforts to cure or attempt suppression of the physiological efforts of the body to cleanse itself. Health is normal and harmonious vibration of the elements and forces composing the human entity on the physical, mental, and moral (emotional) planes of being, in conformity with the constructive principle (great law of life) in nature."

Naturopathy teaches that every cell of the body needs the same three factors for life and health:

- Coordination within a single cell, which is controlled by chemical means, and coordination throughout the entire body by means of hormonal and nervous systems. If this coordination is upset, a state of ill health results.

- Adequate drainage, to rid itself of toxic end products of metabolism. Without adequate drainage, the health of cells is negatively impacted.

- Nutrition in form of the right balance of proteins, carbohydrates, and fats, and the vitamins, minerals, and essential fatty acids.

Naturopathic medicine uses many therapeutic modalities to prevent illness and heal the body, including botanical medicine (herbs), homeopathy, dietary modifications, nutritional medicine, fasting, hydrotherapy, spinal manipulation, physiotherapy, and massage.

For example, one form of hydrotherapy prescribed by naturopathy is cold foot baths. This is a simple hydropathic technique, one of many which are intended to channel the body's vital energies in the direction of improved health and well-being. A variant described by naturopathic practitioners is "Morning Dew Walks," walking barefoot on the wet, dewy grass each morning. This is said to provide the same tonic and refreshing effects on the body as cold foot baths.

*Usefulness*—Naturopathy is a broadly-based system of natural healing useful for the prevention and treatment of a wide range of health problems.

*Research*—In *Traditional Medicine and Health Care Coverage,* naturopathic medicine was recommended as a system that could be beneficial as an adjunct to conventional systems of health care.

*Comparisons*—Naturopathy can be compared to other systems of natural healing, such as Ayurveda and traditional Chinese medicine. In its use of spinal manipulation, it shares some concepts with chiropractic. In its application of herbs to health problems, it is comparable to herbal medicine.

*Conditions or illnesses best suited for*—Naturopathy is best for bringing the healing power of nature to focus on a patient's conditions and in strengthening the immune system for greater resistance to disease.

## Orthomolecular Medicine

Nutritional medicine considers that health problems begin when the body's chemical balance is thrown off. It attempts to rebalance this chemical state and restore wellness using only substances that occur naturally in the body. These are primarily vitamins, minerals, and other nutrients that are known to be essential or beneficial to health. Dr. Linus Pauling, a Noble Prize-winning chemist and physicist, coined the word orthomolecular medicine for this nutritional approach; *ortho* meaning normal or correct. His intent was to provide the body with the right balance of nutrients to create normal, or above normal, health.

It was Dr. Pauling's belief that vitamins' health-fortifying properties became even more potent in larger doses. In large enough doses, Pauling felt vitamins gave an enormous boost to the body's ability to resist the stress and heal the ravages of illness, along with preventing many major diseases from cancer to liver damage. This stress on using large doses of vitamins led to orthomolecular medicine becoming known as megavitamin therapy.

The United States government's recommended daily allowance (RDA) of these vitamins and other nutrients only represents the minimum quantity needed to prevent dietary deficiencies. Practitioners of orthomolecular medicine believe that to engender true health, we need to go far beyond the RDA in our daily consumption of vitamins, minerals, and other beneficial substances. For example, the RDA for vitamin C is 60 mg per day, the minimum amount necessary to prevent scurvy. However, for optimum health and vitality, Dr. Pauling recommends much higher levels of vitamin C—from 2.3 grams to 10 grams daily—"for the preservation of good health and the treatment of disease." Dr. Pauling even believes that due to individual differences for many people, the optimum daily dose may be from 250 mg to 20 g or more. One of the most universal recommendations is the taking of antioxidant supplements for maintaining good health, building up the immune system, and reducing the risks of heart disease and cancer.

In fact, vitamin C is one vitamin with health benefits that orthomolecular medicine particularly endorses. In its view, the intake of this vitamin needs to be very large to keep the immune system working at optimum.

*Usefulness*—Any condition that can benefit from the right dosages of vitamins, minerals, and increased physical vitality.

*Research*—An article in *Orthomolecular Psychiatry*, entitled "The Method of Determining Proper Doses of Vitamin C for the Treatment of Disease by Titrating to Bowel Tolerance" demonstrated that adjusting the dose of vitamin C in relation to its laxative effect could determine the correct doses for treating flu and the common cold.

The British medical journal *Lancet* published a paper on "Prevention of Neural Tube Defects: Results of the Medical Research Council Vitamin Study." The study showed the importance of the B-complex vitamin folic acid in preventing birth defects. A deficiency in folic acid in women of child-bearing age can cause a condition known as spina bifida, in which the spinal column of the child is malformed, causing paralysis. Other research has shown that women in this group need to have adequate levels of folic acid before they become pregnant, as by the time it is determined they are pregnant, it is too late to add the nutrient for preventive effect. For this reason, certain foods, breads, and grains are being fortified with folic acid. The recommended dietary allowance for folic acid is 400 mcg per day.

The *American Journal of Clinical Nutrition* in a study entitled "Beta-carotene and Cancer Prevention: The Basel Study," showed that some cancers had lower rates of incidence when higher levels of beta-carotene, which is converted in the body into vitamin A, are present. Other research has shown there are as many as four hundred different carotenes, many of which may have similar preventive properties.

*Practitioners*—Orthomolecular ideas are now gaining acceptance in the conventional medical community as an essential tool in treating disease, and many physicians practice it under the title of nutritional medicine. Many alternative health practitioners and nutritionists also use megavitamin therapy for maintenance of health and to remedy specific problems.

*Comparisons*—Orthomolecular medicine can be compared to vitamin and mineral therapy.

*Conditions or illnesses best suited for*—Achieving nutritional balance in the body, and treating deficiency-related illnesses; determining someone's individual health needs in reward to the right balance of vitamins, minerals, and nutrients; counteracting the physiological effects of environmental pollution, depletion, and contamination.

## Osteopathy

Osteopathy, like chiropractic, is a medical system that seeks to promote health by manipulating and aligning the body, with special emphasis on the spine. The name comes from the Greek words *osteo* (bone) and *pathos* (disease). Dr. Andrew Still founded the first School of Osteopathy in 1892 in Missouri. He taught and demonstrated that many physical problems were caused from musculoskeletal and spinal disorders, and could be remedied through osteopathic treatment. Osteopathy has been used to successfully treat asthma, high blood pressure, heart conditions, headaches, nerve disorders, and arthritis.

Osteopathy deals primarily with the musculoskeletal system, one of the largest systems in the body, and one of its largest energy consumers as well. Osteopathic holds that bodily structure and function are completely interdependent. If the musculoskeletal system is altered in any way, the body's function immediately alters as well. Conversely, any alteration in body function is believed to set off an immediate alteration in the musculoskeletal system. These alterations can arise from standing of moving wrong, as well as the traumas of daily living.

In America, osteopaths graduate from medical school like all other physicians. Many perform surgery and prescribe drugs just like conventional doctors. However, osteopathic practitioners spend approximately 60 percent of their time working on the back, neck, and other joints. In cranial osteopathy the bones of the skull are gently manipulated. This therapy has helped headache sufferers and those with a range of reversible eye conditions. Infectious diseases have also been treated successfully by osteopathy, possibly because the manipulation of the body restores the flow of lymph through our lymph nodes, with considerable benefit for the immune system.

*Usefulness*—Osteopathy is useful in restoring health to those whose problems arise from incorrect functioning of the musculoskeletal system, including the spinal, cranial, and pelvic areas.

*Research*—An article in the *Journal of American Osteopathic Association* entitled "Manipulative Therapy of Upper Respiratory Infections in Children," reported that children treated with osteopathy for respiratory infections had less negative effects and more rapid rates of recovery from their illness. Benefits were attributed to enhanced blood and nerve supply, and improved functioning of the immune system. An article in the *Journal of the American Osteopathic Association* entitled "Clinical Evaluation of Osteopathic Therapy in Measles," reported more rapid rates of recovery and less negative effects for children with measles who had been treated with osteopathy.

*Practitioners*—Licensed Doctors of Osteopathy (D.O.)

*Comparisons*—Like chiropractic, osteopathy focuses on spinal manipulation as a primary avenue to healing.

*Conditions or illnesses best suited for*—Osteopathy has been shown to benefit spinal, cranial, pelvic, joint, and breathing problems, as well as high blood pressure, heart trouble, arthritis, headaches, and nerve conditions.

## Reichian Therapy

Dr. Wilhelm Reich, a member of Sigmund Freud's inner circle, studied body processes, seeking to learn how to return them to normal functioning. He believed a person's character could be read in their musculature and the way they hold themselves. Reich eventually came to teach that because so many of us hold in our fears, frustrations, stress, and the emotional injuries we suffer, they become locked deep within our musculature. This stiffens the body and restricts the free flow of its vital energies, and is called character armor. Reich also taught that the tension in the body from emotional blocks can affect muscles, internal organs, and blood flow to areas of the body. Reichian therapy uses breathing techniques to locate and release the emotional blocks that create body armor.

"You look for a place where people surrender control, crying, laughing, remembering something." writes Reich. "It can release what has been locked up there for a long time."

Reichian therapist Karla Freeman, L.C.S.W., states, "The artistry and skill of the practitioner is to work with an individual in the moment, as they unfold, and not to supply a technique, but be aware of all these things while you're letting a person see who they are, helping them to find ways to work through what is fearful to them." At the end of a session, people report they can feel the differences between the muscular armor they developed around them, and their body in its natural state.

*Usefulness*—Reichian therapy is useful for people who are anxious and depressed, those suffering from post-traumatic stress, addictions, and sexual and physical abuse. It also helps people get in touch with their emotions, with consequent benefit to intimate and family relationships, and other aspects of their lives.

*Practitioners*—Primarily psychotherapists who have trained at a Reichian institute.

*Conditions or illnesses best suited for*—Opening people up who are out of touch with or overwhelmed by their feelings.

## Traditional Chinese Medicine (TCM)

Traditional Chinese medicine could also be described as the Taoist view of health and longevity. Many of the principles are surprisingly modern, including an emphasis on preventive health, nutrition and diet, herbal remedies, exercise, breathing techniques, and a concern for the total physical, mental, emotional, and spiritual well-being of the individual.

The word *Tao* is pronounced *dao* as in Dow Jones. It means path or way. Simply stated, the Tao is the right path through life for a particular individual. The ideogram for Tao is made up of symbols for head on the right side, and walk on the left and bottom of the character. It indicates a way of life guided by the mind rather than the body.

Traditional Chinese medicine holds that life depends on three elements, called the Three Treasures (san bao) which function together as a single organic unit if health and vitality are to be preserved. The Three Treasures are:

- Essence (jing)

- Energy (chi)

- Spirit (shen)

Jing, also translated as vitality, is the state of our physical body and all of its constituents, especially the essential bodily fluids. Chi is the primal life force, touching every cell and organ of the body and energizing its vital functions. Shen then refers to the processes of the mind; thought, feeling, will, and intent, and awareness and cognition.

As stated in the *Wen-tzu Classic* from the first century B.C., "The body is the temple of life. Energy is the force of life. Spirit is the governor of life. If one of them goes off balance, all three are damaged. When the spirit takes command, the body naturally follows it, and this arrangement benefits all Three Treasures. When the body leads the way, the spirit goes along, and this harms all Three Treasures."

Traditional Chinese medicine has always regarded diet and nutrition as the first line of defense against disease. In this sense, many recipes of classical Chinese cuisine serve as prescriptions for health and longevity, and the Chinese kitchen can be seen as the family health clinic. As far back as the seventh century A.D., the Chinese physician Sun Ssu-mo wrote that, "A truly good physician first finds out the cause of the illness, and having found that, he first tries to cure it by food. Only when food fails does he prescribe medication."

An example of traditional Chinese medicine's approach to healthy eating is pearl barley and brown rice porridge, which makes a great wake-me-up at breakfast. Use a cup of brown rice, half a cup of pearl barley, and eight dates. Simmer slowly with seven cups of water for about one and a half hours. Flavor with a few drops of Chinese sesame oil. Add any healthy fruits you desire, such as bananas for potassium. The pearl barley is 17 percent protein. The brown rice provides dietary fiber, B vitamins, and other nutrients. The dates are for energy and nerves.

Chinese medicinal formulas, primarily herbal in nature, are numerous and the varied medicinal formulas are somewhat complex, so you will need to find a good herbalist to advise you on their uses.

*Usefulness*—Traditional Chinese medicine is considered to remedy a wide range of physical problems. Herbal supplements in the form of tonic broths, teas, and drinks, as well as exercise and breathing are all prescribed in the treatment of chronic illnesses.

*Research*—There are numerous research papers available on traditional Chinese medicine. An article in the *Journal of Traditional Chinese Medicine* entitled "Application of traditional Chinese drugs in comprehensive treatment of primary liver cancer," revealed Chinese medicine and conventional Western medicine make a particularly potent combination. Liver cancer patients found too weak to undergo conventional chemotherapy and surgical procedures were given Chinese herbal potions. After a few months, most regained enough strength to proceed with chemotherapy and surgery, and recuperate without undue difficulty afterward.

*Comparisons*—With its emphasis on diet, exercise, and herbal therapies, traditional Chinese medicine can be compared, in principle, to Ayurvedic medicine, Western nutritional regimes, and naturopathy.

*Conditions or illnesses best suited for*—Traditional Chinese medicine is effective against almost all human illnesses. It is particularly useful in the treatment of chronic disease.

## Visualization Therapy

Visualization therapy, also called imagery or guided imagery, from its applications in sports and performance medicine, has now become an important tool in Western medicine and psychotherapy, endorsed by alternative and conventional health professionals. Hundreds of studies have shown that visualization can play a potent role in enhancing wellness, and it has an especially large impact on the immune system.

One of the pioneers of visualization is Carl Simonton, M.D., a radiation oncologist and founder of the Simonton Cancer Centers in Pacific Palisades, California (see Chapter 7). He teaches cancer patients to focus the mind's extraordinary forces for healing on their illness via the lens of visualization. Patients are shown how to develop imagery based on their own unique psychology and then marshal it on behalf of their own well-being. One man who overcame his cancer, visualized it as little black balls and his body's healing powers as a stream of water the size of a firehose which washed them relentlessly away. The visualizations that Dr. Simonton's patients used tended to be symbolic and dramatic. Knights in armor on white horses, for example, might rush at cancer cells with their spears to systematically destroy them. The visual and emotional power of these images may have given a further boost to the healing process and heightened the effect of visualization on the body's processes.

- The book *Getting Well Again* reports that despite all the potential for individual variations research indicates that effective images generally contain the features listed below. Because imagery is highly individual, what is pointed out are the significant qualities of the symbols, not the symbols themselves.

- The cancer cells are weak and confused.

- The treatment is strong and powerful.

- The healthy cells have no difficulty repairing any slight damage the treatment might cause.

- The army of white blood cells is vast and overwhelms the cancer cells.

- The white blood cells are aggressive, eager for battle, quick to seek out the cancer cells and destroy them.

- The dead cancer cells are flushed from the body naturally and normally.

- By the end of the imagery, you are healthy and free from cancer.

- You see yourself reaching your goals in life, fulfilling your life's purpose.

In some forms of visualization, the therapist supplies the imagery instead of the patient (known as guided imagery). One physician who does this is psychiatrist Gerald Epstein, who has developed specific visualizations to deal with specific health problems. Visualization, he says, is simply the mind thinking in pictures. "Mental imagery, like intuition, is a type of non-logical thinking. Logical, discursive thinking is used for making contact with people in the everyday world and with what can be called objective reality. Mental imagery is the thinking used for making contact with our inner subjective reality. The language of images is commonly experienced as night dreams or day-dreams. Anyone familiar with imagery learns almost immediately that we can work with this language as easily as we can work with spoken language. Indeed, the ability to understand and communicate in the language of images probably precedes the ability to communicate with words. Becoming aware of the language of images requires only that we turn our attention to it."

Author and psychotherapist Adelaide Bry also recommends the use of preconstructed scripts to direct. "The very best visualization for healing you can program is one that comes from your inner being. It is really up to you to discover what only you know: why you have 'dis-ease' and how you can again create body/mind-ease. All scripts should be preceded by inducing a state of deep relaxation and visualizing a place that you've experienced as beautiful and peaceful."

Here are brief examples of some healing visualizations:

- *Visualize healing energy circulating through and soothing the illness*—This energy might appear as golden or white light, or in another form you recognize as healing. If your energy is low and you're feeling tired, depressed, weak, or chilled, breathe in energy from imagined sunlight. If you're feeling hyperactive and restless, see your excess energy flowing out through your feet into the ground. If you suffer from a physical condition that heat can help, visualize and feel warmth in the sick or injured area. This facilitates the flow of blood with its healing properties to the area.

- *Visualize the healing process*—This can be either symbolic or based on images from medical texts. Transform what you know about healing your illness—its location, how it affects that part of the body, whether it involves the skin, muscles, an organ, or bodily system—into a positive image. Visualize the disease healing itself and the part of the body it affects is becoming better. Basic sensations of the healed state you may want to incorporate into your visualization are: smoothness, comfort, gentle warmth, suppleness of new tissues, moistness, resiliency, strength, and vitality.

- *Visualize a state of wellness*—Picture the sick or injured part of your body as completely healed and your whole person as radiantly healthy. See yourself as you wish to be: bursting with vitality and energy, at your healthiest, filled with positive feeling about your life. Visualize yourself walking in the sunshine in this marvelous state of health, in tune with life. Know that the potential for this state lies within you right now, just beneath the symptoms that mask your wellness. In the mystical tradition there are many variations on the theme of seeing the self immersed in a brilliant white light representing the universal energy which is our life force.

*Usefulness*—Visualization is useful in creating a positive mental and emotional state in which the immune system can function at its most effective. Visualization and imagery have been found beneficial in the treatment of cancer and other health problems, including the common cold.

*Research*—There is an extensive body of research attesting to the effectiveness of visualization in mind/body medicine. The journal *Psychosomatic Medicine* published an article entitled "Behaviorally Conditioned Immunosuppression" showing that visualization and imagery boost the immune system paving the way for health and healing.

*Comparisons*—In the way it harnesses the mind's power for stress relief and to promote wellness and healing, visualization can be compared to meditation techniques.

*Conditions or illnesses best suited for*—An important aid in healing from all forms of injury or illness.

## Yoga

Yoga has been defined as a discipline focusing on posture, musculature, consciousness, and breathing. The purpose of yoga is to promote mental and physical well-being through healthy development and maintenance of the physical body. The main practices are asanas, or cleansing postures, and the pranayama, or breathing techniques. Yoga, too, believes a majority of physical ailments come from tension and mental factors.

Yoga originated in India some two thousand years B.C. The word *yoga* is Sanskrit for union and can also mean to join or integrate. The most popular form of yoga in America, where five million or so people practice yoga, is Hatha yoga, or physical yoga. Many Western health professionals routinely recommend yoga as part of their treatment regimens for many serious illnesses, and it is often taught to outpatients in clinics and hospitals. Hatha yoga is divided into three disciplines: breathing techniques, exercises and postures, relaxation practices.

Yoga teaches that nasal breathing controls the flow of prana, a vital life force similar to the chi vital energy of Chinese medicine. Breathing, it is believed, connects the mind and emotions through the parasympathetic nervous system, and reduces tension, so through breathing correctly, negative emotions such as anger, frustration, and depression can be controlled. Stretching, another important component in yoga, helps people to get in touch with their body. In conjunction with breathing this can trigger the beneficial chemical and hormonal reactions of body relaxation response, a key tool in protecting the body from the ravages of stress.

Yoga has traditionally been used for flexibility, relaxation, and meditation. But, recent studies show that yoga also confers aerobic benefits, as well as improved stamina, balance, and coordination. Medical research also indicates the practice of yoga may benefit the immune system, which benefits a variety of physical and mental ailments.

*Usefulness*—Yoga is both a mental and physical therapy. Yoga has helped those suffering from anxiety, depression, and other mental conditions.

*Research*—The *Yoga Biomedical Trust Survey* asked those who practiced routinely if they felt yoga had benefited their condition. More than 90 percent of respondents claimed it had helped them recover from conditions such as alcoholism, anxiety, back pain, cancer, duodenal ulcers, heart disease, and muscle disease.

The journal *Neuropsychobiology* published a paper on the subject of "Changed Pattern of Regional Glucose Metabolism During Yoga Meditative Relaxation," indicating that a patient's dependency on insulin for the treatment of diabetes can be reduced through yoga.

In the *Journal of Mental Deficiency Research*, a study on "The Integrated Approach of Yoga: A Therapeutic Tool for Mentally Retarded Children: A One-Year Controlled Study," found retarded children who were taught yoga showed improvements in social adaptation and in intelligence quotient.

*Practitioners*—Yoga is taught worldwide, and can be adapted to users from children to senior citizens. Yoga instructors advertise in local newspapers, yellow pages, and often teach classes through local houses of worship.

*Comparisons*—Yoga can be compared to the breathing and physical exercises taught and used in traditional Chinese and Ayurvedic medicine.

*Conditions or illnesses best suited for*—Yoga is a good choice for stress reduction, as it combines stretching, breathing exercises, and meditation.

# *A Guide to Natural Remedies for Ailments*

*T*his chapter presents suggestions drawn from the various alternative therapies for treating nearly twenty-five common ailments and conditions. As always, the emphasis in nearly all of these treatments is on tapping into the body's natural ability to heal itself by helping boost its vitality and immune functioning. The remedies given here are those that are easiest to use.

## *Basic Nutritional Support*

Before examining the remedies, here are recommendations for basic nutritional support. To get well, and stay well, you need to give your body the raw materials it needs to rebuild and maintain your vitality at optimum levels. Here is a daily vitamin and mineral program that most nutritionists and other alternative therapists, and many conventional physicians, can agree will work well with natural remedies.

You can also take a multi-vitamin/mineral capsule if you can find a good formula that contains the following nutrients. Be sure to check the label for dosage, as some require several capsules a day to achieve the stated potencies.

## DAILY DOSAGES OF NUTRITIONAL SUPPLEMENTS

| Nutrient | Quantities |
| --- | --- |
| Magnesium | 200–300 mg |
| Selenium | 100–200 mcg |
| Zinc (picolinate) | 30–50 mg |
| Amino acids | One serving, protein powder |
| Vitamin A | 10,000–25,000 IU |
| Vitamin B1 | 50–100 mg |
| Vitamin B5 | 100–200 mg |
| Vitamin B6 | 50–200 mg |
| Vitamin B12 | 100–1,000 mcg |
| Folic acid | 400 mcg |
| Niacin | 100–200 mg |
| Coenzyme Q-10 (Ubiquinone) | 30–60 mg |
| Vitamin C (Calcium Ascorbate is less acidic than ascorbic acid, will not bother the enamel on your teeth, and will give you some calcium.) | 3,000 mg per day, in three divided doses of 1,000 mg each. Doses can be divided further if desired. |
| Vitamin E (d–Alpha Tocopherol and mixed tocopherol concentrate. Natural sources.) | 400 IU |

## Alzheimer's Disease

Eliminate all potential sources of aluminum. Be sure not to use aluminum cookware.

Consult Chapter 8, "The Mind, the Immune System, and Healing," for brain tonics and nutrients which may delay or prevent the onset of Alzheimer's disease. Genetics may be a factor in this disease, but bad diet most certainly plays a role as well.

## Burns

Medical experts suggest gently applying apple cider vinegar on a sunburn or any other type of minor burn every few hours can help reduce pain.

Tea Tree oil, a botanical from Australia, applied to the skin is useful for relieving pain and promoting healing. Aloe vera, squeezed directly from the cactus-like plant or used in the form of a gel can also relieve pain and promote healing.

> **MEDICAL NOTE**
>
> *The suggestions for treatments in this chapter are not intended as a substitute for consulting your physician. Please remember that all matters regarding your health require medical guidance and supervision and are your responsibility to obtain.*

Vitamin E applied to the burn can help the healing process and prevent scarring.

## Cancer

While there are natural ways to assist in the prevention and healing of cancer, anyone who has cancer or its symptoms should seek professional medical attention immediately, and not delay while using any of the diet and herbal suggestions shown here. They are meant to address some of the beneficial aspects of nutrition that may be of help in complementing proper medical supervision.

### Diet Therapy

The National Academy of Sciences reports that 60 percent of cancers in women and 40 percent of cancers in men may be due to dietary and nutritional factors. For this reason, diet needs to be considered in the prevention and treatment of cancer. An anticancer diet should support the immune system, which is the main defense against cancer and other diseases.

Freshly made juices are nutrient rich (see the section on juice therapy in Chapter 12). Always include some cruciferous vegetables in your meals, like cabbage, broccoli, Brussels sprouts, turnips, and kale. The glucosinolates in these vegetables help neutralize and excrete some of the carcinogens in the environment. Omega-3 fatty acids, like fish oils and flaxseed oils, have been demonstrated to reduce the growth rate of breast tumors.

Eliminate all the foods shown to be connected with cancer. These include nitrates, nitrites, food additives, smoked foods, hydrogenated vegetable oils (trans-fats) including margarine, and excess sugar. Fat intake is a key dietary risk factor linked to cancer, as is a more moderate intake of animal protein. Make sure the meat you buy is hormone free.

Herbs that are particularly helpful in fighting cancer are Pau D'Arco, ginseng, echinacea, green tea, astragalus, garlic and mushroom extracts like shiitake, reishi, and maritake. Use abundant amounts of ginger root, onions, and garlic, which have been demonstrated to contain cancer fighting compounds.

## The Common Cold

The common cold is really a number of conditions which result in similar symptoms. Alternative medical traditions often treat symptoms only, though even this approach can sometimes prevent the condition from worsening.

### Ayurvedic Remedy

An Ayurvedic remedy for colds is ginger tea. Ginger tea is warming and drying, and helps reduce the symptoms of a cold. Take about an ounce of ginger root, then peel and slice thinly. Place in a quart of water and boil until the water is half gone. When the tea has cooled sufficiently to drink, add $1/2$ to 1 full teaspoon of honey to a cup. Honey has a drying effect. You can drink several cups of ginger tea daily for as long as your cold lasts.

### Infection Fighting Foods

New research underscores the idea that whole foods, especially fruits and vegetables, are especially effective in fighting the common cold.

They contain thousands of disease fighting compounds (phyto-chemicals) that boost the efficacy of the food's vitamin content.

According to Charles B. Inlander and Cynthia K. Moran who made a study of the subject in *77 Ways to Beat Colds and Flu*, there are lots of foods that can help you fight the common cold. Here are some of them:

- *Bell peppers*—Help the immune system fight colds, asthma, bronchitis, and respiratory infections; high in vitamin C.

- *Blueberries*—Block the attachment of bacteria-causing chemicals; curb diarrhea and antiviral activity; high in natural aspirin.

- *Carrots*—Boost the immune system, fight infection, and contain the beneficial antioxidant beta-carotene.

- *Chili peppers*—Contain capsaicin, a phytochemical compound that acts as a painkiller, alleviating headaches. Chili also contains antibacterial agents and antioxidants, and opens the sinuses and other air passages, breaking up mucus in the lungs, and preventing bronchitis.

- *Cranberries*—Have strong antiviral, antibiotic properties, and an unusual ability to prevent infectious bacteria from sticking to cells lining your bladder and urinary tract.

- *Garlic*—Actions are antimicrobial, antifungal, and suitable for a wide range of infectious conditions.

- *Mushrooms (Asian, including shiitake)*—A great antiviral flu treatment containing antiviral compounds that aid immune functions.

- *Mustard (including horseradish)*—Acts as a decongestant/ expectorant, breaking up mucus in air passages.

*Foods for Congestion*
- *Onion (including shallots, yellow, red, not white)*—Powerful anti-inflammatory, antiviral, antioxidant with a strong

phytochemical sedative; fights asthma, chronic bronchitis, infections.

- *Pineapple*—Antiviral among other healing attributes; has enzyme that suppresses inflammation.

- *Plum*—Antiviral, laxative.

- *Raspberry*—Antiviral, high in natural aspirin.

- *Soybean*—Active antiviral agent.

- *Strawberry*—Antiviral.

- *Tea (including black, oolong, and green, but not herbals)*— Ingredient catechin makes it antibiotic, antidiarrheal, antiviral.

- *Yogurt*—Boosts immune response, spurs activity of killer cells that attack viruses; a cupful daily reduces colds, other upper respiratory infections in humans; helps prevent and cure diarrhea.

*Chinese Herbal Remedies for Colds, Flu, and Fever*
According to Daniel Reid and *The Complete Book of Chinese Health and Healing* the following are known as effective formulas for treating the common cold:

- *Bi Yan Pian (nose inflammation pills)*—Effective against head colds caused by wind-heat or wind-cold invasion, including sneezing, watery eyes, sinus congestion, and related headache. Also good for chronic rhinitis, sinusitis, hay fever, and general mucus congestion in the face. Should be taken immediately upon contracting a cold.

- *Ching Chee Hua Tan Wan (clean air tea)*—This is a classical prescription for clearing phlegm and heat from the lungs, throat, and sinuses. It remedies congestion and excess phlegm in the bronchial passages and sinuses and provides relief for chronic asthma and emphysema. This formula is most effective for chronic conditions and the later stages of serious colds that have become entrenched in the respiratory system, not for the early stages of external wind invasion.

- *Gan Mao Ling (common cold tablet)*—An excellent remedy for common cold and flu, including chills, fever, swollen lymph glands, sore throat, stiff neck and shoulders. Sedates excess heat and dispels external wind invasions, both hot and cold. May be used in higher doses to cure colds, lower doses to prevent colds.

- *Yin Chiao tablets (honeysuckle and forsythia tablets)*— Effective remedy for colds with heat symptoms, such as flu, sore throat, swollen lymph nodes, fever, headache, stiff neck, and shoulders. Expels toxins by inducing sweating. To be effective, it must be taken on the first day that symptoms appear, and continued for two or three days.

### Orthomolecular Remedy (Vitamin C)

Dr. Linus Pauling, a Nobel Prize winning chemist, had this to say about the common cold. "It is wise to carry some 1,000 mg tablets of ascorbic acid with you at all times. At the first sign that a cold is developing, the first feeling of scratchiness of the throat, presence of mucus in the nose, or muscle pain or general malaise, begin the treatment by swallowing two or more 1,000 mg tablets. Continue the treatment for several hours by taking an additional two tablets or more every hour."

### Folk Medicine Remedies

The three Rs of folk medicine are resistance to disease, repair of injury, and recovery from illness. Here are some folk remedies for coughs and colds, tested and used in Vermont by D.C. Jarvis, M.D.

- *Old fashioned cough remedy*—Boil one lemon slowly for ten minutes. This softens the lemon so more juice can be gotten out of it, and also softens the rind. Cut the lemon in two and extract the juice with a lemon squeezer. Put the juice into an ordinary drinking glass.

Add two tablespoons of glycerine, two tablespoons equal one ounce. Stir the glycerine and lemon juice well, then fill up the drinking glass with honey.

If you have a coughing spell during the day, take one teaspoonful. Stir with a spoon before taking. If you are apt to be awakened at night by coughing, take one teaspoonful at bedtime and another during the night. As the cough gets better, lessen the number of times you take it.

• *Honeycomb treatment*—Honeycomb is excellent for treating the breathing problems that accompany colds. Honeycomb soothes the lining of the entire breathing tract. Eat some of the waxy comb substance from which all the honey has been extracted every day. In addition to chewing the comb, eating honey each day is also part of the treatment. For this purpose, comb honey is the first choice, but if for any reason comb honey is not available, a tablespoon of liquid honey as a dessert with each meal will still help ameliorate cold symptoms.

• *Nasal sinusitis treatment*—When inflammation of one or more of the sinuses appears, it generally develops on an alkaline-urine-reaction background. When honeycomb is chewed, the urine reaction is shifted from alkaline to acid, showing how quickly honeycomb brings about a change in body chemistry. The amount of honeycomb for one chew can be gauged by the ordinary chew of gum. Take one chew of honeycomb every hour for four to six hours. Chew each amount for fifteen minutes and discard what remains in your mouth. If the sinus attack is acute, these four to six chews should bring about a disappearance of the symptoms in one-half to one day's time. The nose will open up, the pain will disappear. Body energy will return and the sinuses will return to normal.

- *Aromatherapy treatment for colds and flu*—Aromatherapist Roberta Wilson says the essential oils of plants can help to fight colds and flu in two ways. First they can ward off illness or hasten recovery by boosting immunity. Second, they can ease many of the discomforts of colds and flu when used in baths, chest rubs, compresses, and inhalants.

- *Cold and flu fighting bath*

      1 drop marjoram oil
      1 drop myrrh oil
      2 drops elemi oil
      3 drops lemon oil
      3 drops tea tree oil

Disperse the essential oils in a bathtub filled with warm water. Soak in the bath for twenty to thirty minutes, taking care not to become chilled. Repeat as necessary.

- *Cold and flu chest rub*

      1 drop ginger oil
      1 ounce carrier oil
      2 drops frankincense oil
      2 drops rosemary oil
      2 drops thyme oil
      3 drops eucalyptus oil
      4 drops pine oil

Place the carrier oil in a clean container, add the essential oils and blend. Massage the oil over your chest and back several times daily until your symptoms subside. If you have any questions about using an essential oil blend, check first with a qualified aromatherapist or your physician.

## Cold Sores

- Alternative medical practitioners recommend: Let zinc lozenges dissolve on the lesion.

- To prevent cold sores, try avoiding foods rich in arginine, like nuts, seeds, cereal, grains, and chocolates.

- Tea tree oil, applied with a cotton tip, will kill viruses on contact and rapidly heal some cold sores.

## Depression

Many cases of depression require outside help. If necessary, get in touch with an appropriate specialist. However, a compilation of sources follows:

- Low blood sugar, or hypoglycemia, is a common cause of depression. Cut sugar from the diet. Avoid simple carbohydrates, processed, and refined foods. Eat a diet high in complex carbohydrates and fiber. Don't use artificial sweeteners.

- Cut out alcohol and smoking. Limit caffeine intake to one beverage a day.

- Take chromium 100 mcg three times a day.

- Food allergies can cause depression. Avoid foods that cause your allergies.

- Walk briskly in nature 30–45 minutes a day and do other exercises as much as possible.

- Depression has been linked to deficiencies in the B-complex group, especially to thiamine (B1). B-complex vitamins are water soluble, and usually destroyed in cooking. A supplemental B vitamin tablet once a day may be helpful, along with foods rich in B vitamins. Potassium and magnesium phosphate act as a nerve tonic and liver cleansing herbs help metabolize toxins contributing to depression.

- Avoid sleeping too much. If you live in a northern latitude, get checked for SAD (Seasonal Affective Disorder). In addition to regular daily supplements take melatonin 2 mg at bedtime during the dark months. If your symptoms are seasonal, add amino acid tyrosine 500 mg one or two capsules three times daily; amino acid D-phenylalanine 500 mg one or two capsules three times daily.

- The herb St. John's wort is used worldwide as a mood lifter. It is available in dried or liquid form. Follow the directions on the label, and take note of the fact that taking St. John's wort can increase your sensitivity to sunlight, so measures should be taken to protect yourself from sun exposure while taking this herb.

- The herb ginkgo biloba, made from the leaves of a long living tree, have been shown to be helpful for depression and improved mental function. Follow the directions on the label, which generally call for one 60 mg tablet of ginkgo biloba in the morning and one in the evening. Siberian ginseng is another herb that can be helpful in depression. The amino acid phenylalanine is found in sunflower seeds, black beans, watercress, and soybeans. Tryptophan, a feel good amino acid, can be found in sunflower seeds, pumpkin seeds, and evening primrose seeds.

## *Ear Infections*

Immediately consult a physician for ear infections. You doctor may recommend the following:

- Use acetaminophen (as in Tylenol) for pain relief.

- Elevate the head of the bed to facilitate draining of tubes to relieve pressure. Use a warm compress to the ear to relieve pain.

- Drink plenty of fluids.

- Take a dropperful of echinacea dissolved in a glass of water three times a day. This is considered safe for adults and children over a year old. Adults can also take echinacea capsules and drink echinacea tea.

- For children with chronic ear infections, determine if the child has a food or inhalant allergy. Food allergens can include wheat, eggs, dairy foods, corn, citrus, and peanut butter. In babies, breast feeding as long as possible will help prevent development of allergies, as the baby receives protection from the mother through the milk. Don't let a baby drink from a bottle while lying down, as the fluid can collect in the ear. While breast feeding, try to keep the baby's head raised, for the same reason. While you have a cold or ear infection, greatly reduce or eliminate sugars from your food.

## Fingernail Problems

The most frequent cause of fingernail problems is exposure to weather and household chemicals. Vitamin and mineral deficiencies can show up as problem nails. To protect your fingernails, which in turn protect the delicate nerve endings at the end of your fingers, wear rubber gloves when you are working with water or chemicals. Moisturize your hands with an aloe vera cream. Consume adequate protein in your diet, as a rule; eat an amount the size of a deck of cards with each meal. If you do not get enough protein, your hair and fingernails will not grow normally.

## Glaucoma

Glaucoma, an eye disease that can lead to blindness, occurs in two forms, acute and chronic. Acute glaucoma is a medical emergency that requires immediate medical attention.

Chronic glaucoma accounts for 90 percent of cases. People over age forty-five, or who have a family history of glaucoma, should have an eye exam with a glaucoma test annually. There are natural remedies that can help reduce elevated eye pressure, and in some cases bring it back to normal. Glaucoma is not an inevitable effect of aging and heredity. For example, in parts of Africa, where glaucoma was epidemic, researchers found that improved nutrition was a much better cure for glaucoma than drugs. Whether you have glaucoma or are at risk of developing the disease, you may benefit greatly from a daily program of nutrients and supplements, and a healthy diet as described in Chapter 1.

- As a natural remedy for glaucoma, take part in a regular exercise program.

- Avoid the use of corticosteroids when possible. Consult your physician on this medication.

- Don't smoke. Avoid secondhand smoke.

## Heart Attack

The American Heart Association tells us that eleven million people have a history of heart attack or angina. Each year one and a half million people will have a heart attack. By applying the right kind of exercise, nutrition, and care, the risk of heart attack can be reduced. Most coronary heart disease is the result of the narrowing of the coronary arteries by a buildup of fatty plaques on the inner surface of these arteries, which narrow the opening and obstruct blood flow, a condition known as atherosclerosis. Reducing cholesterol levels in the blood is one of the most important ways to prevent this problem. Foods associated with lower cholesterol levels include soy lecithin, oat bran, olive oil, yogurt, apples, carrots, garlic, and chili peppers.

### Exercise Treatment

Exercise on a daily basis will also effectively lower cholesterol. A Baylor College of Medicine Study demonstrated that daily and vigorous exercise is one of the best means of lowering blood cholesterol, ridding the body of excess fats, and increasing the ratio of HDL (good) cholesterol in relation to LDL (bad) cholesterol.

### Vitamin Supplements

A new study shows how women can protect their hearts. A study of a large number of women nurses has shown that a high intake of folic acid and vitamin B6 appears to reduce, by almost half, a woman's risk of a heart attack. Both folic acid and B6 are B-complex vitamins. The study suggests that higher levels of the two vitamins can be obtained from foods and supplements; foods including fruits, vegetables, and whole grains. In regard to supplements, the study, published in the *Journal of the American Medical Association,* suggests that the current RDA for these vitamins, which is 180 mcg for folic acid and 1.6 mg of B6, is inadequate to provide maximum protection against heart disease. The greatest amount of cardiac protection in the study was achieved with daily intakes of more than 400 mcg of folic acid and more than 3 mg of B6. The vitamins were protective whether obtained from food or supplements.

Dr. Eric B. Rimm, of the Harvard School of Public Health, who directed the study, says, "Everyone should be at two to three times the RDA for folic acid and B6 to achieve the maximum reduction in risk. The exciting news is that a substantial reduction in risk can be achieved easily, without a dramatic change in diet. You don't have to give up everything you eat. You just have to eat more foods like fortified cold cereals, orange juice, spinach and other leafy greens, whole grains, bananas, potatoes, chicken, and fish."

This was the first study to show a direct link between folic acid and vitamin B6 and the prevention of heart disease. Over a period of 14 years, the women who consumed the most folic acid were one-third less likely to suffer a heart attack than those who consumed the least folic acid. Those who consumed the most vitamin B6 were 33 percent less likely to have a heart attack then were those who consumed the least. Those with the highest consumption of both vitamins reduced their coronary risk by 45 percent.

In addition, another important discovery in the control of plaque formation in the arteries was made when an amino acid, homocysteine, was identified as a causative factor when it is present at elevated levels. Studies have linked high levels of homocysteine in the blood to a greatly increased risk of suffering a heart attack. Homocysteine is believed to increase coronary heart risk by damaging cells that line the arteries, causing blood clots, and narrowing blood vessels by promoting growth of smooth muscle cells. Homocysteine is normally present at low levels in the bloodstream, and the object is to keep it low. Fortunately the answer is in certain nutrients. Folic acid, along with vitamins B6 and B12 are known to help control homocysteine.

Vitamin E is good for the heart. As an antioxidant it helps control the activity of free radicals. In addition, it works to prevent abnormal platelet aggregation. Recommended dosage for vitamin E is 400 IU per day up to age forty and 800 IU per day over age forty. Minerals considered necessary for healthy heart functioning are magnesium, calcium, chromium, copper, selenium, and zinc.

An antioxidant compound, alpha lipoic acid, helps prevent heart disease by reducing the damage to cholesterol carrying lipoproteins. Richard A. Passwater, Ph.D. reports that through its metabolic activities, alpha lipoic acid can lower total cholesterol levels by as much as 40 percent.

Furthermore, Coenzyme Q10 (Ubiquinone) generally known as CoQ10, has been shown to be an important nutrient in keeping the heart healthy. According to James F. Balch, M.D., and Phyllis A. Balch C.N.C., Coenzyme Q10 appears to be a giant step forward in the treatment and prevention of cardiovascular disease. A six-year study at the University of Texas found that patients being treated for congestive heart failure who took CoQ10 in addition to standard therapy achieved a 75 percent chance of survival after three years compared to a 25 percent survival rate for those solely using conventional therapy. A study by Japan's Center for Adult Diseases in collaboration with the University of Texas found that CoQ10 supplementation lowered high blood pressure even without medication or changes in diet. In heart failure, supplements of CoQ10 are believed to help the remaining muscle cells to do their jobs more efficiently. The nutrient is found in all foods, but is easily destroyed by cooking and processing. The body's levels of CoQ10 drop after age twenty-five.

Many heart patients are very low in CoQ10. Deficiencies were found in 75 percent of patients undergoing surgery. Dr. Peter

Langsjoen, a cardiologist, says, "in 80 percent of my heart patients, I see a clinical improvement within four weeks of administering Coenzyme Q10." The supplement is a vegetarian product derived from biological fermentation. The recommended dosage is 30 mg per day or as directed by your health consultant.

### Alcohol

The previously mentioned nurses' study also demonstrated the protective effect of drinking moderate amounts of alcohol. The women who consumed the most folic acid, and who had at least one alcoholic drink a day had a 75 percent lower risk of suffering a heart attack than those who consumed the least amount of folic acid and who drank no alcohol. The researchers said they expect the findings in the nurses' study will also apply to men.

### Herbal Remedies

An herbal supplement, Hawthorn berries, is considered one of the most effective heart tonics. It has been shown to speed recovery from a heart attack, lower blood pressure, regulate the heart beat, and strengthen the heart muscle. Hawthorn berries come in capsules of 455 mg each, and can be taken two to three times daily. It is also available in liquid form as a standardized extract of 1 percent flavonoids.

## Hypertension (High Blood Pressure)

Hypertension, or high blood pressure, is a serious health problem that requires medical attention. It is called the silent killer because it damages many organs without causing pain. Medical science has identified two types of hypertension, primary and secondary. Primary hypertension has no known cause. Secondary hypertension is brought about by an identifiable cause, such as kidney disease. When the identifiable cause is treated, the blood pressure returns to normal. The following recommendations are for primary hypertension.

- As a natural remedy for hypertension, if you are over-weight, lose weight. This change alone can sometimes lower your pressure into a normal range. Even losing ten pounds can make a difference. Lower the amounts of saturated fats (meats and dairy) in your diet.

- Find out if you are salt sensitive. If sodium is affecting your blood pressure, eliminate it from your diet. If you reduce sodium, increase your intake of potassium-rich foods like eggplant, peas, pears, and peppers.

- Eat a high fiber diet.

- Follow an exercise program, brisk walking in nature is excellent.

- Use stress management techniques (See Chapter 6, "Stress and Distress"). Don't smoke.

## Indigestion

Indigestion concerns problems in the upper gastrointestinal tract, which includes the esophagus, stomach, and gallbladder. Heartburn is one of the usual symptoms; gas, bloating, and belching are other symptoms. Common causes are ulcers, lactose intolerance, heartburn, hiatal hernia and esophagitis, food allergies, gallbladder disease, H. pylori, and candidiasis. Lesser known causes are deficiency of either hydrochloric acid or pancreatic enzymes.

- First see your physician to rule out the above diseases, including cardiac trouble, as possible causes.

- Over age sixty, over half the people in that group have low gastric acidity. A doctor can determine this with a diagnostic test. There is also a self test you can perform at home for low gastric acidity. Take a tablespoon of apple cider vinegar or lemon juice when you are experiencing indigestion. If this eliminates your symptoms, then you may be deficient in stomach acid. If it makes your symptoms worse, you have an overproduction of stomach acid. If the vinegar helps, you can take it with meals, sipping it with a little water or using it as a salad dressing.

- If you are deficient in pancreatic enzymes, you will have trouble when you eat fatty foods. This may cause belching or bloating or a feeling of fullness an hour after a fatty meal, or you may feel ill. Your physician may suggest that you reduce your intake of saturated fats (meats and dairy). If you lack pancreatic enzymes you can take supplements, which are sold in health food stores. These contain pancreatic enzymes from animal sources, and may include bromelain, which is made from pineapples. The enzymes in papaya are also helpful. When starting a meal, eat enzyme-rich foods like melons and fresh juice first.

## Insomnia

If you have trouble staying asleep during the night, or are waking up too early, you have a problem with insomnia causing sleep deprivation, which can affect your health and efficiency.

### Things You Can Do

- Try aromatherapy for insomnia. Add eight drops of lavender or marjoram essential oil to your bath water, or place four drops of either on your pillow.

- A gentle massage of your neck and shoulders before bedtime can help you sleep. This can be a self-massage if you wish. Take ten minutes of massage. You can use an aromatherapy lotion base as a massage cream. Use about a half ounce of lotion base and add seven drops of an individual oil or combination of oils. Lavender is calming and sedative, alleviates stress, and is an immune builder. Marjoram's warm and sedative properties ease physical tension, stress, and insomnia. Aromatherapy essential oils and lotion base are available at health food stores. Be sure to follow the directions on the labels.

- When it comes to using imagery, think of a night when you wanted to sleep, but couldn't. See yourself struggling to stay awake and longing for a chance to sleep. Then just let yourself go and fall asleep. Try this imagery in bed, just before you want to sleep.

### Juices

Fresh juices deliver a lot of nutrients quickly. With the help of a juicer you can try some of these combinations:

- *Broccoli, tomato, and carrot*—Sources of niacin.

- *Celery and carrots*—One stalk of celery, and two raw carrots with the greens removed. Juice and drink one hour before bedtime.

- *Grape and pineapple*—High in glucose and sucrose.

- *Lettuce and celery*—Traditional remedies for insomnia. Juice three to four lettuce leaves and one stalk of celery.

- *Parsley, collard greens, and blackberries*—Sources of magnesium.

- *Spinach, carrots, and peas*—Sources of vitamin B6.

### Other Food Therapy

- *Milk or turkey*—Both contain the amino acid L-tryptophan, which induces sleep.

- *Niacin, magnesium, and vitamin B6*—All are co-factors in the conversion of the amino acid tryptophan into the sleep-inducing chemical serotonin.

- *Melatonin capsules*—Have helped many people get to sleep. They supplement the natural secretions of the pineal gland, which decrease as we age. Capsules are taken about thirty minutes before you want to sleep. The capsules come in various strengths, from less than 1 mg to 3 mg. The amount of melatonin needed increases with age. Some people do fine with just 0.2 mg. Some put three drops of liquid melatonin under their tongue and sleep well. Follow the directions on the label, and take note of the warning you see there. Melatonin is not to be taken by pregnant or lactating women, individuals with autoimmune conditions or depressive disorders, or children under age sixteen. Also, do not take melatonin when driving a motor vehicle or operating machinery.

- *Valerian*—Is the best known herb for insomnia, and has the property of reducing activity in the central nervous system. Follow the directions on the label. For a combination of sleep herbs, select one that combines chamomile, balm, hops, oats, passionflower, and valerian.

## Jet Lag

Jet lag is that out of sync feeling you get when you have crossed one or more time zones. As a remedy for jet lag establish a regular routine, including regular bedtime and rising time, at least two days before your journey. Whenever possible, fly during the day instead of at night. Drink lots of fluids on the airplane and avoid diuretics like coffee and tea. Don't drink alcohol on the airplane. Get out into the sun when you arrive. Keep up an exercise routine.

### The Anti-Jet Lag Diet

This diet was developed by Dr. Charles Ehret of the Argonne National Laboratory. It has been used by the U.S. military to prevent jet lag during troop movements, and is reportedly effective in doing so. Determine your breakfast time at your destination on the day of arrival. Feast-fast-feast-fast on home time: Start three days before departure day.

- *On day one*—Feast eat heartily with a high protein breakfast and lunch and a high carbohydrate dinner. No coffee except between 3 and 5 P.M.

- *On day two*—Fast eat light meals of salads, light soups, fruits, and juices. Again, no coffee except between 3 and 5 P.M.

- *On day three*—Feast again.

- *On day four*—Fast, departure day. If you drink caffeinated beverages, take them in the morning when traveling west or between 6 and 11 P.M. when traveling east. Going west, you may fast only half the day.

Sleep until the normal breakfast time at the destination, but no later. End your final fast at breakfast time at your destination. Feast on a high protein breakfast. Stay awake and active. Take the rest of the day's meals at the mealtimes of your destination.

In general, feast on high protein breakfasts and lunches to stimulate the body's activity cycle. Selections can include eggs, hamburgers, steak, high protein cereals, and similar foods.

Feast on high carbohydrate suppers to stimulate sleep. Supper selections can include spaghetti and other pastas, with no meatballs or meat sauces; also no potatoes, other starchy vegetables, and sweet desserts.

Fast days deplete the liver's store of carbohydrates and prepare the body's clock for resetting. Suitable food choices include: fruit, light soups, broths, skimpy salads, unbuttered toast, and half pieces of bread. When fasting, try to keep carbohydrates and calories to the minimum. Enjoy your journey, and have many happy landings.

## Leg Cramps

Leg cramps that occur at night can be both annoying and painful, and can interfere with your sleep. It is possible that prescription drugs can cause cramping, so check with your doctor on possible side effects of any prescriptions you are taking. Some diuretics taken for hypertension or heart problems can cause an imbalance in potassium and magnesium in the bloodstream. A blood test will determine this, and the right mineral supplements can give relief from the symptom.

Leg cramps are most commonly caused by a calcium deficiency. There is a continuing problem with calcium deficiency in the population, especially among women. By supplementing your diet with calcium you can prevent both leg cramps, and a much more serious problem, osteoporosis. Nutritionists recommend adding nonfat yogurt and skim milk to your diet. Remember that sugar and caffeine reduce the absorption of minerals, calcium in particular.

Medical experts suggest the following:

- Eliminate as much sugar and caffeine from your diet as possible.

- Take 1,200 mg of calcium at bedtime, preferably in a ratio with magnesium. Pregnant women should check with their doctor beforehand.

- Vitamin E 400 IU (natural) twice a day for two weeks. If symptoms are relieved, reduce the dosage to 400 IU once a day. If the symptoms come back, the dosage can be increased until symptoms are relieved, but never take more than 1,200 IU of vitamin E daily.

- Supplements of magnesium 400 mg a day; vitamin A 10,000 IU daily, and potassium 100 mg per day if you are not already doing so.

## Motion Sickness

Ginger offers relief from seasickness, or motion sickness, a problem that originates in the inner ear. The reaction of the body is to produce an overabundance of hormones that precipitate the dizziness and nausea of motion sickness. A natural remedy for this problem has been found in ground gingerroot capsules, which are sold in health food stores. Ginger tea, made by steeping peeled and chopped fresh ginger in boiling water, or iced ginger tea are also good remedies. In studies at Purdue University by Dr. Varro Tyler, Professor of Pharmacognosy, ginger was found more effective than some popular over-the-counter motion sickness remedies and without the side effects of the OTC preparations.

Begin your travel day with a small, low fat, starchy meal. Skip fatty, greasy foods before and during your journey. Stay as still as possible on the ship, car, or airplane. Get fresh air. Don't read. Use stress management techniques to relieve anxiety. Keep your mind occupied. Take two or three ground gingerroot capsules before traveling and additional capsules every three to four hours. You can buy candied ginger, available at Asian food markets, and chew on it while you are traveling or drink ginger tea. The tea can be drunk hot or cold. Iced ginger tea is the recommended beverage for boating crews and passengers.

## Osteoporosis

Half of all American women over age fifty will suffer a broken bone caused by osteoporosis sometime in their lives. One in every five victims of the disease is male. Osteoporosis, or loss of bone density, causes bones to thin, making them more likely to break. The latest research shows that supplements can stop bone erosion completely. If you are over age fifty-five, you can keep your bones strong by consuming the amount of calcium contained in three glasses of milk every day, and by taking other preventive measures. Medical experts also recommend the following:

- Eat more calcium-rich foods, which include low fat or non-fat yogurts and dairy products. Collard greens, spinach, and sardines (with the bones in) are also good sources. Intake of protein should be limited to six ounces daily, and salt should be used sparingly. Avoid sugar, alcohol, and caffeine.

- Do not smoke. Exercise regularly.

- Add the following supplements to your diet:
  Boron 2 mg per day
  Calcium citrate 1,200 mg at bedtime
  Magnesium 400 mg a day
  Vitamins, a good multiple vitamin with 400 IU of vitamin D

If osteoporosis is a serious problem for you, you should consult your physician and discuss possible drugs that may work in conjunction with nutritional support.

## Overweight

Correct food choices and exercise are still the best ways to lose weight. Most people gain their excess weight by eating too much of the wrong foods and exercising too little. The answer is not in a restrictive diet, but in a change to a healthier lifestyle. Making this change should make diets and drugs unnecessary. Nutritionists agree with the following:

- Start with whole foods, use whole grains, fruits, and vegetables. Keep your daily fat intake to 25 percent or less (about 45 to 50 grams.) Add foods that have a significant amount of fiber. You need about 25 grams of fiber a day to keep your system running well. Insoluble fiber, from fruits, whole grains and vegetables makes you feel full without adding to your weight. It also helps with elimination, and is a preventive against colon cancer and other problems. Barley, legumes like dried beans, and whole oats are good sources of insoluble fiber, which act to lower cholesterol and block excess fats from entering your system. It is best to get your fiber from whole grain, rather than in a bran that has been removed from the whole grain. If you eat enough whole foods, you won't need bulk products like psyllium husks.

- Drink lots of pure water, distilled or reverse osmosis purified. Water helps you lose weight. Cut down on alcohol, which the body treats as a fat.

- If you limit your fat intake to 20 to 25 percent of calories-as-fat, you can hope to keep weight in check. A study of women at Cornell University, who were allowed to eat as much as they wanted, with just the one requirement that they eat low fat foods in that 20 to 25 percent of calories-as-fat range, showed that they lost weight on these food choices. You can eat large amounts of vegetables, on a ratio of 60 percent raw and 40 percent cooked, and still lose weight. Vegetables and fruits are diffuse foods, meaning

they are full of water. Start the day with fresh
vegetable juice, which has less sugar than fruit juice.

- Above all, avoid refined sugars, known as simple
carbohydrates. Refined and processed foods are not
conducive to weight management, or to good health
in general. They are a large part of the problem.

- The kind of exercise that includes slow, sustained
effort such as brisk walking, is good for weight loss.
Take at least one brisk walk for forty-five minutes to
an hour every day. It will give you aerobic benefits
and help increase your metabolic rate, which burns
excess calories.

Correct food choices and exercise are still the best way to
healthy weight management.

## Prostate Problems

Just beneath the bladder, only in men, is the prostate gland. About
the size of a walnut in normal health, it is capable of enlarging to
the size of an orange. The problem is the prostate encircles the
prostatic urethra, the tube by which urine exits the bladder.
Enlargement in the prostate gland can therefore result in more frequent trips to the bathroom, especially at night, along with a sensation of needing to urinate.

- A doctor's examination may include a blood test for PSA,
prostatic specific antigen. A digital rectal examination, a
DRE, is quick and painless, and allows the doctor to actually feel the prostate. Your doctor may also order other
tests, such as urinalysis or an ultrasound scan. Prevention is
the best way to deal with the prostate, and a yearly medical
examination is a good start on the prevention program.

- Fortunately, there are a number of alternative methods that
can be used to care for the prostate, under medical care

and with the approval of your doctor, that can complement medical supervision. One of the more common prostate problems is BPH or benign prostatic hypertrophy. In this case, which can be detected in a medical examination, the prostate becomes enlarged. By the time they turn fifty, approximately 30 percent of all men will begin to notice some difficulty in urination due to BPH. In approximately 60 percent of men over age fifty the prostate becomes enlarged.

- Diet and nutrition can help with prostate problems. The mineral zinc, found in sunflower seeds and pumpkin seeds, has been shown to be helpful in shrinking an enlarged prostate. You can supplement your diet by taking 30 mg of zinc per day, 2 mg of copper per day, 400 IU of vitamin E, 1,000 mg of vitamin C and one tablespoon (or three capsules) of flaxseed oil per day. The mineral selenium and carotenes, such as beta-carotene, should be added for their antioxidant effects.

- Avoid high fats and foods high in animal fats, especially red meats. Cut down or eliminate your intake of refined sugar. All of the above have been linked to a higher incidence of prostatic cancer.

- For BPH, an herbal preparation made from the berries of the saw palmetto plant has been shown in clinical trials, to reduce the size of the prostate and reduce the symptoms. It is available in health food stores. Follow the directions on the label.

- Nettle root extract has been shown to act synergistically in combination with saw palmetto, and is added to some preparations.

- Another herbal, *Pygeum Africanus,* has a long history of use for urinary disorders. Made from the powdered bark of a tree, the active compounds have anti-inflammatory effects, and can promote regression of the symptoms of BPH without toxic side effects.

• Prostatitis is a condition, most frequently seen in men between age twenty and fifty, in which the prostate becomes infected or inflamed. If you have prostatitis, you should see a medical doctor. Maintaining a strong immune system is a preventive strategy, as prostatitis is linked with lowered immunity and a depleted glandular environment. Herbal preparations for prostatitis can include purple cornflower as an anti-infection agent; Pipsissewa which contains arbutin, a urinary tract antiseptic, and stimulates blood flow to the prostate. Horsetail is recommended for helping with acute prostatitis.

> **IMPORTANT!**
>
> If you are experiencing prostate problems or symptoms you should see a medical doctor without delay. Symptoms that require a medical examination include painful urination, lower back pain, pain in the pelvis, fever, and a weak stream of urine. You have the urge to urinate with no result, you get up two or three times a night to urinate, or your bladder still feels full when you finish urinating. The Cancer Association recommends that males over the age of forty receive yearly examinations for the presence of prostate enlargement and cancer.

• A yearly examination for men over age forty, along with the dietary and nutritional recommendations shown above, will go a long way in preventing prostate problems.

## Periodontal Disease

Gum disease is a major problem in the United States. Three out of four adults have some form of the disease. The American Academy of Periodontology estimates that the majority of children have gingivitis, which, if untreated, can cause more serious periodontal disease.

The principal cause of gingivitis is tartar buildup on the teeth. The main preventive treatment is flossing at least once a day, as tooth brushing does not remove the food particles that insinuate themselves between the teeth and the gums. Flossing and professional dental care are preventive measures you can take. A toothpaste containing peroxide and baking soda, which combine to form oxygen, is helpful.

Dr. Paul Keyes, a dentist who pioneered the nonsurgical approach to periodontal disease, recommends the following method of oral hygiene: "Dip your toothbrush in a solution of half hydrogen peroxide, half water, then dip it in baking soda and smear the mixture along the gum line, making sure to get it in all the crevices between the teeth and gums." His office procedures involve a technique for scaling and root planing of the problem area below the gumline. Dentists familiar with Dr. Keyes's techniques can provide this non-surgical treatment.

## Rheumatoid Arthritis

Arthritis is a term that relates to several diseases that affect the joints. Osteoarthritis is the most common form, affecting people mostly over forty-five years of age. Rheumatoid arthritis, unlike osteoarthritis, is a more systemic disease. It can strike people in their twenties. There is evidence that the cause is related to a failure of the autoimmune system, a case where the immune system is fighting the body it is supposed to protect.

- There is now substantial evidence pointing to diet as a major factor contributing to the development of symptoms. One reason for this is that food makes great demands on the immune system. Foods contain a large number of allergens that the body is constantly trying to fight or adapt. Therefore, finding the foods that stimulate symptoms is a logical first step to take. It can take up to three months for this program to take effect. If you want to attempt this, modify your diet to reduce sugar, other refined carbohydrates, and saturated fats including red meat. Increase the amount of fresh fruits and vegetables and whole grains. Avoid foods of the nightshade family for a month to see if you find relief from symptoms. Nightshades include potatoes, eggplant, paprika, peppers, tomatoes, tobacco, and cayenne.

- Eliminate the possibility of food allergies or food sensitivities. Some other foods that cause sensitivities in cases of rheumatoid arthritis are milk and dairy products, corn, wheat, and beef. Eliminate as many animal and vegetable fats as possible, except for fish oils and increase the amount of fish you eat.

- A program of stress management is important. Regular exercise, as can be tolerated, is recommended—pool exercises, swimming, and gentle yoga are suggested exercises. As one yoga teacher put it, "if you can move your body even one inch in any direction, you can benefit from yoga exercises."

## Sore Throat

A sore throat can be the first sign of a cold, the flu, a viral or bacterial infection, or a strep throat infected with streptococcal bacteria. It is important to determine if you have a strep throat. Some of the symptoms are a sudden fever of 102 degrees or more and a red, inflamed throat covered with white patches. If you have any of these symptoms, consult your doctor.

For the average sore throat, which is generally the result of a cold or flu virus, here is a home remedy. Gargle with a mixture of half water and half hydrogen peroxide to help fight infection. Do not swallow this mixture. Gargle with crushed aspirin mixed with water to relieve pain. Drink warm herbal or decaffeinated tea with honey, or sip warm water with honey and lemon. If you have recurring sore throats, especially those associated with ear infections, you might have a food allergy. Natural remedies urge two or more cloves of garlic at the first sign of a sore throat, and two cloves a day until it is cleared up. Dr. Varro Tyler of Purdue University suggests that you brew goldenseal tea, using two teaspoonfuls of the dried herb in boiling water, allow it to cool, and use it as a gargle. Repeat gargles as needed for a maximum of two or three days.

## Tension Headaches

Tension headaches are the most common form of headache and are caused when the sensitive nerve endings in your head and neck are irritated by tense muscles which also press on the blood vessels in your scalp.

- Check to see if your headaches are connected to food allergies or sensitivities.

- Use stress reduction techniques to combat tension.

- Stretch your muscles every half hour, and massage the neck and shoulders. Use an aromatherapy oil of peppermint.

- Use moist heat to relieve pain—take a warm shower or bath or use a moist or dry heating pad on your neck. Engage in regular exercise.

- A cup of coffee constricts blood vessels and boosts the pain-relieving power of aspirin by about one third, according to Fred Sheftell, M.D., a specialist in headache pain.

- Eat meals at regular times and never skip a meal.

- Take a nap, or a brisk walk.

- Add a drop of peppermint oil to facial oil, dilute sufficiently, and apply under nose and behind ears.

## Ulcers

Ulcers form when the mucus membrane lining of the stomach loses its ability to repel the acids of the stomach, which then begin to digest the stomach itself. One in ten men and one in twenty women may expect to have one in their lifetime. Medical science has learned a great deal about ulcers in the recent past. If you have recurring ulcers, you should talk to your doctor about the possibility of an infection of the bacterium Helicobacter pylori, known as H. pylori. Treatment with antibiotics can wipe out the infection in as little as two weeks.

- Susan Lange, O.M.D., recommends the flower essence of dandelion to help people let go of the tension that comes from holding fear in their stomachs.

- Avoid the use of aspirins and other nonsteroidal anti-inflammatory drugs (NSAIDs).

- Avoid smoking, alcohol, and antacids made with calcium carbonate.

- Eat a high fiber diet unless your symptoms are acute, in which case you should avoid roughage and raw vegetables until symptoms are under control.

- David Frawley, O.M.D. recommends the Ayurvedic remedy of aloe vera gel. Take one or two teaspoonfuls three times daily, mixing it with enough honey or a nonacidic fruit juice to improve the taste.

## Varicose Veins

Varicose veins are most often found in the legs, but can occur in the arms as well. In the U.S., nearly 25 percent of women and 10 percent of men have them. The condition is caused when the veins carrying blood from the legs back to the heart become engorged and dilated.

- Julian Whitaker, M.D. recommends 30 grams of fiber a day, and lots of blackberries and cherries, which contain compounds that prevent varicose veins.

- Perform a program of exercise that will contract the leg muscles, such as running, cycling, or walking. Also, take care to relieve standing or sitting for long periods of time by stretching the legs or walking, even briefly. Whenever possible, elevate your legs, ideally with your ankles higher than your hips.

• Maintain an appropriate weight for your proportions, and avoid obesity.

• Eat a high fiber diet with abundant fruits and vegetables. Use a fiber bulking agent if necessary. The idea is to avoid chronic constipation, a major contributing factor to varicose veins.

• Wear support stockings if needed. Before putting on the stockings, lie on your back with hips near a wall and legs perpendicular to the floor to encourage blood flow. Rest in this position for a few minutes, then put on your support stockings. As a hydrotherapy remedy, alternating hot and cold leg baths, about three minutes each, can stimulate circulation in the legs, according to Agatha Thrush, M.D.

## Wrinkle Prevention

Anything that takes moisture out of your skin can cause wrinkles, but the worst offender is the ultraviolet light of the sun. With the more effective sunscreens now available, and a greater knowledge of how the skin works, we have a better chance than ever to prevent wrinkles. One of the primary functions of the skin is to excrete toxins, and some of those toxins can cause blemishes, dryness, and dullness.

• The best way to prevent toxins from reaching the skin in the first place is to drink eight 8-ounce glasses of pure water a day, preferably distilled or reverse osmosis treated water. Drinking adequate amounts of pure water will help prevent dry skin as well.

• Always use sunscreens, as tanning is an enemy of the skin. Use a skin moisturizer, such as an SPF 15 or higher sunscreen on a daily basis, not just for the beach. Don't let sunscreen give you a false sense of security. For long exposures in the sun you need the protection afforded by clothing, hats, and shade.

- Smoking definitely ages your skin prematurely. If you smoke a pack and a half a day you will wrinkle about ten years sooner than a nonsmoker. There are many reasons for this: the effect of nicotine on your system, the smoke that dries on your face, the depletion of vitamin C, the pursing of your lips to inhale and exhale, and the constriction of blood vessels, which affects the nutrients trying to reach the skin.

- For an aromatherapy solution, aromatherapist Victoria Edwards recommends one drop of rose oil and two drops of everlast oil to an ounce of rose hip seed essential oil. Store it in a dark glass bottle and apply it every morning, right after cleansing your skin. Always observe the dilution cautions from your supplier when diluting essential oils.

# Bibliography

Arnott, Robert M.D. *Dr. Bob Arnott's Guide to Turning Back the Clock.* Boston: Little, Brown and Company, 1995.

Anselmo, Peter with James S. Brooks. M.D. *Ayurvedic Secrets to Longevity & Total Health.* Englewood Cliffs, New Jersey: Prentice Hall, 1996.

Bosco, Dominick. *The People's Guide to Vitamins and Minerals.* Chicago: Contemporary Books, 1989.

Brennan, Richard. *The Alexander Technique, Natural Poise for Health.* Rockport, MA: Element Books Limited (England), 1991.

Carper, Jean. *The Food Pharmacy*, New York: Bantam Books, 1989.

Claire, Thomas. *Bodywork.* New York: William Morrow and Company, 1995.

Cooper, Kenneth H., M.D. *Dr. Kenneth Cooper's Antioxidant Revolution.* Nashville: Thomas Nelson Publishers, 1994.

Epstein, Gerald, M.D. *Healing Visualizations, Creating Health Through Imagery.* New York: Bantam Books, 1989.

Inlander, Charles B. and Cynthia K. Moran. *77 Ways to Beat Colds and Flu.* New York: People's Medical Society, 1994.

Khalsa, Dharma Singh, M.D., with Cameron Stauth. *Brain Longevity: The Breakthrough Medical Program that Improves Your Mind and Memory.* New York: Warner Books, 1997.

Jarvis, D.C. M.D. *Folk Medicine.* New York: Galahad Books, 1996.

Lee, William H, R.P.H., Ph.D. *Vitamin Primer*, New York: Lee Press, 1995.

LeShan, Lawrence. *How to Meditate, a Guide to Self-Discovery.* Boston: G.K. Hall & Co., 1974.

Lin, David J. *Free Radicals and Disease Prevention, What You Must Know.* New Canaan, CT: Keats Publishing Inc., 1993.

Lindlahr, Henry. *Philosophy of Natural Therapeutics.* Chicago: Lindlahr Publishing Co., 1919.

Lockie, Andrew Dr. & Dr. Nicola Geddes. *The Complete Guide to Homeopathy, The Principles and Practice of Treatment.* New York: DK Publishing Inc., 1995.

Morgan, Dr. Brian L.G. *Nutrition Prescription*. New York: Crown Publishers, 1987.

Murray, Frank *Ginkgo Biloba*. New Canaan, CT: Keats Publishing, 1993.

Ornish, Dean, M.D. *Stress, Diet & Your Heart*, New York: Holt, Rinehart and Winston, 1982.

Ody, Penelope. *The Complete Medicinal Herbal*. London: Dorling Kindersley, 1993.

Pauling, Linus Dr. *How to Live Longer and Feel Better*. New York: W.H. Freeman and Co., 1986.

Pierpaoli, Walter, M.D., Ph.D, and William Regelson, M.D., with Carol Colman. *The Melatonin Miracle*. New York: Simon & Schuster, 1995.

Reid, Daniel. *The Complete Book of Chinese Health & Healing*. Boston: Shambala, 1995.

Sahelian, Ray, M.D. *DHEA A Practical Guide*. Garden City Park, New York: Avery Publishing Group, 1996.

Stanway, Andrew Dr. *Alternative Medicine, A Guide to Natural Therapies*. London: Bloomsbury Books, 1992.

Trattler, Ross, Dr. *Better Health Through Natural Healing*. New York: McGraw-Hill, 1985.

Tyler, Varro E., Ph.D., "Grape Expectations," *Prevention*. June, 1997.

Weil, Andrew, M.D. *Natural Health, Natural Medicine. A Comprehensive Manual for Wellness and Self Care*. Boston: Houghton Mifflin Co., 1990.

Wilson, Roberta. *Aromatherapy for Vibrant Health & Beauty*. Garden City Park, New York: Avery Publishing Group, 1995.

White, Timothy P., Ph.D. and the editors of the U.C. Berkeley Wellness Letter. *The Wellness Guide to Total Fitness*. New York: REBUS Distributed by Random House, 1993.

Winawer, Sidney J., M.D. and Shike, Moshe, M.D. *Cancer Free, The Comprehensive Prevention Program*. New York: Simon & Schuster, 1995.

Zimmerman, Marcia, M.Ed. "Food As Medicine." *Delicious Magazine*, August 1997.

# *Audiotapes*

Bruyere, Rosalyn L. and Jeanne Farrens. *Chakra Healing*. Los Angeles: Audio Renaissance.

Bry, Adelaide *Visualization: Directing the Movies Of Your Mind,* Los Angeles: Audio Renaissance Tapes 1989.

Collinge, Dr. William. *The Mind/Body Medicine Library: Cancer.* Los Angeles: Audio Renaissance.

Collinge, Dr. William. *The Mind/Body Medicine Library: Heart Disease and Hypertension.* Los Angeles: Audio Renaissance.

Collinge, Dr. William. *The Mind/Body Medicine Library: Stress Reduction.* Los Angeles: Audio Renaissance.

Davich, Victor N. *The Best Guide to Meditation.* Los Angeles: Audio Renaissance.

Goldberg, Philip and Daniel Kaufman. *The Audio Guide to Natural Sleep: A Drug-Free Approach.* Los Angeles: Audio Renaissance.

Hendricks, Gay, Ph.D. *Conscious Breathing.* Los Angeles: Audio Renaissance.

Joy, W. Brugh, M.D. *Healing with Body Energy.* Los Angeles: Audio Renaissance.

LeShan, Lawrence, Ph.D. *The Heart's Code.* Los Angeles: Audio Renaissance.

LeShan, Lawrence Ph.D. *How to Meditate.* An Audio Renaissance Tape Program, Distributed by St. Martin's Press, New York 1987.

O'Connor, Richard, *Personal Meditations, Six Individual Meditations,* Los Angeles: Audio Renaissance Tapes 1990.

Pearsall, Paul, Ph.D. *Superimmunity: A Prescription for Health.* Los Angeles: Audio Renaissance.

Pearsall, Paul, Ph.D. *The Pleasure Prescription: A Prescription for Health.* Los Angeles: Audio Renaissance.

Reilly, Harold J., D.Ph.T., D.S. *Natural Healing by Edgar Cayce.* Los Angeles: Audio Renaissance.

Simonton, O. Carl M.D., *Getting Well,* a two cassette program with a 32 page self help guide

Thurston, Mark. *Meditation by Edgar Cayce*. Los Angeles: Audio Renaissance.

Watts, Alan W. *Alan Watts Teaches Meditation*. Los Angeles: Audio Renaissance.

Winawer, Dr. Sidney J. and Nick Taylor. *Healing Lessons*. Los Angeles: Audio Renaissance.

Young, Shinzen. *Five Classic Meditations*. Los Angeles: Audio Renaissance.

For more information about Audio Renaissance Tapes, to request the complete Audio Renaissance Catalog, or to order tape programs, call: 800-452-5589.

## Internet Health Sites

You can search the forum databases for a topic of your choosing.

### America Online Health Forums

- Baby Boomers (Keyword: "Baby Boomers")
  a forum for all of you that were born between 1946 and
  1964. In the section on Baby Boomer Issues you'll find
  discussion groups like these: Single Again/In Midlife,
  Losing a Parent, Empty Nesters, Stay-at-Home Fathers,
  New Age Thoughts, Prozac/Zoloft, Fitness for Boomers,
  Endometriosis and Infertility.

  The Boomer Roll Call board has a group on weight loss,
  and there is a support group for menopause, which is
  called "Power Surge."

- Parents Information Network (Keyword: "PIN")
  has resources and support groups for parents.

- Longevity Online (Keyword: "Longevity")
  Articles on anti-aging medicine, alternative medicine, and
  other health topics from past and present issues of
  *Longevity* magazine. The Forum has a Health Exchange, a
  message board for topics in the magazine.

### Multimedia Self-Care Showcase

This is an illustrated encyclopedia of health, medicine and lifestyle
information. Included is a listing of searchable databases, in each
of them is a similar encyclopedic listing of the topics: Alternative
Medicine, Home Medical Guide, Lifestyles & Wellness, Mental
Health & Addictions, Human Sexuality, Informed Decisions,
Health Reform & Insurance, Men/Women/Children's Health,
Senior's Health and Caregiving.

### Special Interest Message Boards in the Better Health & Medical Forum

There is a list of message boards you can browse through, representing a wide range of special interest topics. Each board has postings from AOL members who share that interest. For starters, try the board for Alternative Healing Approaches, where you will find a long list of topics on the subject of alternative medicine. Then click on the board for Diet, Exercise & Fitness. But with all this netsurfing, remember to exercise as much as you can, not only in cyberspace, but in the real aerobic world where you live.

*More Internet Resources*

- Alternative Medicine
  Usenet: Newsgroup: misc.health.alternative

- American Lung Association Homepage
  http://www.lungusa.org

- Anatomy Teaching Modules
  http://www.groups.dcs.st
  http://www.ac.uk/~history/

- Ask Dr. Weil
  http://ogi.pathfinder.com/@DfiHegcACgGHcfkz/drweil/
  Andrew Weil, M.D. answers questions viewers have sent in previously. Web site (http://www.drweil.com)

- The Black Health Net
  http://www.blackhealthnet.com

- Cancer News on the Net
  http://www.cancernews.com

- Clinical Photograph Library
  http://www.njet.com/~enbbs/photo/photo.html

- Complementary Medicine
  http://galen.med.virginia.edu/~pjb3s/complementary home page.html

- Good Health Web
  http://www.social.com/health/

- Health & Exercise
  Usenet:Newsgroup:misc.fitness

- Heartinfo: Heart Association Network
  http://www.heartinfo.org

- Herbal Resources
  http:www.mtsu.edu/~j henry/my herb.html

- Holistic Healing; List Name: holistic
  listserv@siucvmb.bitnet

- Medicinal Herb Garden
  http://www.nnlm.nih.gov/pnr/uwmhg/

- Mental Health Infosource
  http://www.mhsource.com

- Nutrition
  Newsgroup:sci.med.nutrition

- Virtual Library of Medicine, An Index of Links to
  Medical Servers on the Internet
  http://golgi.harrad.edu/biopages/medicine.html

- Yahoo Health Line
  http://www.yahoo.com/health/

### *Medical Journals on the Internet*

- International Journal of Psychiatry, British based research
  journal
  http://www.cityscape.co.uk/users/ad88/psych.htm

- The Journal of Family Practice
  http://www.jfp.msu.edu

- Alternative Medicine Digest
  http://www.alternativemedicine.com

- The Lancet, British Weekly
  http://www.thelancet.com

- New England Journal of Medicine On-Line
  http://www.nejm.org

*Health Web Sites*

- Health on the Net Foundation, Geneva based group that rates and certifies health sites. http://www.hon.ch/home.html

- Metanoia Guide to Internet Mental Health Services http://www.metanoia.org/imhs

## Directory of Alternative Medicine Resources

This directory includes alternative resources we have located in the course of researching and writing this book. They are listed by discipline. Inclusion in the resources listings does not constitute an endorsement or recommendation from the author or the publisher, Renaissance Books. We recommend that you choose all of your health practitioners with care, and upon good local references.

### Acupuncturists

Acupuncture seeks to harmonize energy flow by inserting very thin needles into acupuncture points located on the meridians of the body. The best needle technique is to use sealed and sterilized needles that have been prepackaged, and to discard the needles after one use. Needles are left in place from one second to one hour according to the condition and the acupuncturist's method of treatment.

- Linda King, L. Ac.
  *(Acupuncture, nutrition and herbs, homeopathy)*
  261 Alisal Rd. Suite C-2
  Solvang, CA 93463

- Kathryn Connors L. Ac., N.C.C.A.
  *(Acupuncture, oriental medicine, Chinese herbs, Shiatsu acupressure massage)*
  Solvang, CA 805-569-3370

- Joseph S. Acquah, O.M.D. L. Ac.
  *(Acupuncture, Chinese herbal medicine, tai chi chuan)*
  1273 Westwood Blvd., Suite 205
  Los Angeles, CA 90024
  310-444-0936

- Abayomi Meeks, O.M.D.
  *(Acupuncture, herbal therapy, qigong, tai chi chuan, and its South African counterpart, Isinaphakade Samathonga, Ukolemeleza—South African massage—and Ukuzonga—South African diet therapy)*
  Moyo Associates, Inc.
  1648 Gaylord St.
  Denver, CO 89206
  303-377-2511

- Courtney Witherspoon, L. Ac.
  *(Acupuncture, herbs, polarity, homeopathy, and nutrition)*
  RPP P.O. Box 1266
  New York, NY 10037
  212-491-7433

- The American Association of Acupuncture and Oriental Medicine
  433 Front St.
  Castasauqua, PA 18032
  610-433-2448

*Aromatherapy*

Aromatherapy involves the use of essential oils of plants, a highly concentrated essence diluted in a carrier oil, to treat ailments, and to positively affect emotions and the mind.

- Abena Asantewaa, Ph.D.
  *(Uses aromatherapy as an adjunct to psychotherapy. Inner Light Products)*
  P.O. Box 64
  Berrien Springs, MI 49103
  616-641-5499

- L'dia Muhammad
  *(Aromatherapy and music therapy for a soothing birthing experience)*
  P.O. Box 3256
  Berkeley, CA 94703
  800-782-3999

- Marcia White
  *(Personalized skin care)*
  1415 Old Northern Blvd.
  Roslyn, NY 11576
  516-621-5402

- Aromatherapy Institute & Research (AIR)
  P.O. Box 2354
  Fair Oaks, CA 95628

### Ayurvedic Medicine

Ayurveda, a system of natural healing from India, is truly holistic in that it sees the individual as an integrated whole. Ayurveda, which means "science of life" or "knowledge of lifespan" includes the mental, physical, emotional, and spiritual sides of the person.

- American School of Ayurvedic Sciences
  10025 NE 4th St.
  Bellevue, WA 98004
  206-453-8022

- Canadian Association of Ayurvedic Medicine
  P.O. Box 749 Station B
  Ottawa, Ontario, Canada K1P 5P8
  613-837-5737

- The Chopra Center for Well Being
  7630 Fay Avenue
  La Jolla, CA 92037
  619-551-7788, 888-424-6772

*Brain Longevity*

- Dharma Singh Khalsa, M.D.—Physician, Author, Speaker—
  Alzheimer's Prevention Foundation
  11901 E. Coronado
  Tucson, AZ 85749
  520-749-8374, Fax: 520-749-2669
  www.Brain-longevity.com
  E-mail: Drdharma@aol.com

*Cancer Counseling*

- Simonton Cancer Center
  P. O. Box 890
  Pacific Palisades, CA 90272
  310-457-3811, 800-459-3424

- The Wellness Community
  National Office
  10921 Reed Hartman Highway, Suite 215
  Cincinnati, OH 45242
  513-794-1116, 888-793-WELL, Fax: 513-794-1822
  www.brugold.com/wellness.html.
  E-mail: wellnessnational@fuse.net.

*Chiropractors*

Chiropractic works on the principle that total health is directly
affected by the alignment of the spinal column. Illness and discomfort are the result of misalignment of the spine. Treatment is
centered on adjusting the spine manually to unblock flow of blood
and energy to the nervous system. Treatment can include diet and
nutritional advice, and counseling on the management of stress
and on relaxation.

- The American Chiropractic Association
  1701 Clarendon Blvd.
  Arlington, VA 22209
  703-276 -8800, 800-986-4636

*Dolphin Healing*

- Sabine Eden, R.N., B.A.
  *(Guided swimming with wild dolphins in Hawaii)*
  P.O. Box 783
  Los Olivos, CA 93441
  805-686-9285

*Herbal Medicine*

- The American Herbalists Guild
  P.O. Box 1683
  Soquel, CA 95073

- American Botanical Council
  P.O. Box 201660
  Austin, TX 78720
  512-331-8868

*Hypnotherapy*

- Sabine Eden, R.N., B.A., Clinical Hypnotherapist
  P.O. Box 783
  Los Olivos, CA 93441
  805-686-9285

- The American Institute of Hypnotherapy
  1805 East Garry Avenue, Suite 100
  Santa Ana, CA 92705

- International Medical and Dental Hypnotherapy Association
  4110 Edgeland, Suite 800
  Royal Oak, MI 48073
  313-549-5594, 800-257-5467

*Mind/Body Therapy*

Mind/body therapy brings thoughts and emotions into the healing process. It is practiced by many alternative and conventional medical professionals.

- Ronald W. Davidson, M.D.
  *(Integrates conventional medicine and alternative methods, including acupuncture, ethnic diets, and herbs)*
  1378 President St.
  Brooklyn, NY 11213
  718-756-4523

- The Hale Clinic
  *(Conventional medicine integrated with acupuncture, aromatherapy, chiropractic, Ayurvedic medicine, Chinese herbal medicine, and homeopathy)*
  7 Park Cres.
  London W1N 3HE United Kingdom
  011-44-71-631-0156

- The Progressive Pain Relief and Medical Health Center
  5576 Mayfield Rd.
  Lindhurst, OH 44124
  216-771-5855

- Michael E. Casselberry, M.D., LMT and Ronald B. Casselberry, M.D.
  *(Acupuncture, applied kinesiology, nutritional counseling and homeopathy)*
  Simonton Cancer Center
  P. O. Box 890
  Pacific Palisades, CA 90272
  310-457-3811, 800-459-3424 Fax 310-457-0421
  Tapes and literature 800-338-2360
  http://www.simontoncenter.com.
  E-mail:simonton@lainet.com.

- Andrew Weil, M.D.
  *(Monthly newsletter and other information available)*
  P.O. Box 457
  Vail, AZ 85641

- The American Holistic Medical Association
  4101 Lake Boone Trail, Suite 20
  Raleigh, NC 27606
  919-787-5181

- The Center for Mind/Body Studies
  5225 Connecticut Ave. Northwest, Suite 414
  Washington, D.C. 20015
  202-966-7338

- The Center for Applied Psychophysiology
  Menninger Clinic
  P.O. Box 829
  Topeka, KS 66601
  913-273-7500 Ext. 5375

- Mind-Body Clinic
  New Deaconess Hospital
  Harvard Medical School
  185 Pilgrim Rd.
  Cambridge, MA 02215
  617-623-9530

### Massage

Massage relieves stress, increases blood flow, releases endorphins, and soothes sore muscles, among other benefits.

- Sabine Eden, R.N., B.A.
  *(Shiatsu, acupressure, intuitive feeling)*
  P.O. Box 783
  Los Olivos, CA 93441
  805-686-9285

- American Massage Therapy Association
  820 Davis St., Suite 100
  Evanston, IL 60201
  312-761-2682

- The Rolf Institute
  P.O. Box 1868
  Boulder, CO 80306
  93030 449-5903, 800-530-8875

- The Trager Institute
  33 Millwood
  Mill Valley, CA 94941
  415-388-2688

- International Institute of Reflexology
  P.O. Box 12462
  St. Petersburg, FL 33733
  813-343-4811

- American Oriental Bodywork Association
  6801 Jericho Turnpike
  Syosset, NY 11791
  516-364-5533

- Associated Bodywork and Massage Professionals
  28677 Buffalo Park Rd.
  Evergreen, CO 80439
  800-862-7724

### Meditation

Meditation is a method used by many mind/body, stress reduction and relaxation, and psychoneuroimmunology therapies.

- Institute of Transpersonal Psychology
  P.O. Box 4437
  Stanford, CA 94305
  415-327-2066

- Mind-Body Clinic
  New Deaconess Hospital
  Harvard School of Medicine
  185 Pilgrim Road
  Cambridge, MA 02215
  617-632-9530

- Institute of Noetic Sciences
  P.O. Box 909
  Sausalito, CA 94966
  415-331-5650

### Naturopathy

Naturopathy is an ancient natural system of healing, going back to Hippocrates in the fifth century B.C. It emphasizes the body's ability to heal itself, given the right conditions, foods, and nutrients. It is believed that these healing conditions will be found in nature. Methods include hydrotherapy, homeopathy, herbal medicine, nutrition, spinal manipulation, massage, and physiotherapy.

- The American Association of Naturopathic Physicians
  2366 Eastlake Ave. E., Suite 322
  Seattle, WA 98102

- Ontario Naturopathic Association
  60 Berl Ave.
  Etobicoke ONT M8Y 3C7, Canada
  416-503-9554

### Osteopathy

Osteopathic physicians are licensed medical doctors. They use manipulation of the spine, muscles and bones, and connective tissue to diagnose and treat illness and injury. The focus is on preventive medical care.

- The American Osteopathic Association
  142 East Ontario St.
  Chicago, IL 60611
  312-280-5800

- The American Academy of Osteopathy
  3500 DePauw Blvd.
  Indianapolis, IN 46268
  317-879-1881

### Reichian Therapy

- Karla Freeman, L.C.S.W., Reichian Therapist
  211 E. Carrillo Street, Suite 205
  Santa Barbara, CA 93101
  805-969-2738

### Traditional Chinese Medicine

Traditional Chinese medicine places an emphasis on preventive measures, nutrition and diet, herbal remedies, exercise, breathing techniques, and a concern for the total physical, mental, emotional, and spiritual well-being of the individual.

- American Association of Acupuncture and Oriental Medicine
  4101 Lake Boone Trail, Ste. 201
  Raleigh, NC 27607
  919-787-5181

*Yoga*

Yoga has been defined as a discipline focusing on posture, musculature, consciousness, and breathing. The purpose of yoga is mental and physical well-being through mastery of the physical body.

- International Association of Yoga Therapists
  109 Hillside Ave.
  Mill Valley, CA 94941
  415-383-4587

- Himalayan Institute of Yoga, Science, and Philosophy
  RRI Box 400
  Honesdale, PA 18431
  800-822-4547

# Glossary

*Aerobic Fitness:* The ability to take in oxygen from the air and transport it efficiently to the organs and cells of the body. Aerobic comes from the Greek word for "with oxygen."

*Acupuncture:* The principle is that there is a nervous connection between skin surface at acupuncture points and the internal organs. The stimulation of these points with very fine needles is believed to modify the point, and in so doing, have an effect on other parts of the body.

*Adaptogens:* Naturally available plants and foods that can help maintain good health.

*Ama:* The Sanskrit word for residual impurities in the body. To Ayurvedic physicians it is a sticky substance that blocks body channels and prevents the flow of biological energy.

*Antioxidants:* Vitamins, minerals, and other substances that prevent damaging oxidation of body cells by free radicals. Vitamins C and E, beta-carotene, which the body converts into vitamin A, and zinc are primary antioxidants, along with foods and phytonutrients.

*Aromatherapy:* The method of using naturally distilled essences of plants to achieve positive changes in health.

*Asanas:* Postures or positions used in the Ayurvedic health program to stimulate the circulatory system.

*Ayurveda:* A natural health system from India, where it has been practiced for over 3,000 years. Ayurveda means "science of life."

*Bioflavonoids:* Natural substances found in the leaves, stems, flowers, fruits, and roots of most plants. Abundant in cherries, citrus fruits, buckwheat, and other foods. Work well when combined with vitamin C, calcium, and magnesium.

*Breath Control:* The technique of breath control that is important in aerobic fitness, relaxation, and meditation. Conscious breath control can be learned and practiced, as in Complete Deep Breathing and Yogic Breath Control.

*Bach:* Bach remedies are herbal preparations developed by Dr. Edward Bach, a bacteriologist who worked in London hospitals. He devised approximately 38 herbal remedies based on herbs placed in water. A diluted solution of the water is then taken by the patient.

*Biofeedback:* A method of controlling a system by reinserting it into the results of its past performance.

*Body Mass Index:* A measure of body composition arrived at by dividing your weight in kilograms by the square of your height in meters.

*Carotenes:* Protective chemicals found in vegetables colored orange, red, and dark green. Antioxidants and anti-cancer properties. Best known is beta-carotene, but there are more than 500 carotenoids.

*Chi:* A term used in traditional Chinese medicine and acupuncture therapy to mean "vital energy." Chi is the force that moves every system of the body, both conscious and autonomic.

*Chi Gong:* (also spelled chi kung.) In TCM this is "energy work," which generates vital energy and rejuvenates the body by establishing soothing biofeedback between the nervous and endocrine systems.

*Chiropractic:* A skill by which skeletal joints are manipulated by hand in order to improve and balance the functions of the body.

*Chlorine:* A chemical added to drinking water supplies as a disinfectant. Advisable to remove by filtration or distillation prior to drinking or bathing.

*Cruciferous:* A group of vegetables including broccoli, cabbage, and kale. Counteract the destructiveness of carcinogens in the environment.

*DHEA:* A hormone, dehydroepiandrosterone, that is made by the adrenal glands and can be purchased as a supplement. Supplement is made primarily from wild yams.

*Doshas:* Ayurvedic categories of human behavior each containing a combination of elements—vata, pitta, and kapha.

*Flexibility:* The ability to move limbs, joints, and connective tissue in a good range of motion for your age and condition. Stretching and exercise help to maintain this element of fitness.

*Free Radicals:* Unstable oxygen molecules, submicroscopic particles that dart through the cells of the body like jalopies in a destruction derby, crashing into other particles, cells and tissues. Unstable molecules have an unpaired electron. This makes them reactive—a free radical. They will take an electron from a previously stable molecule, causing a chain reaction of destructiveness. Medical experts consider them central actors in most human health problems.

*Ginkgo biloba:* An herb associated with improved memory, clear thought, and focus.

*Hatha Yoga:* A form of yogic posturing (asanas) used to better one's health.

*Herbal Medicine:* A worldwide system of using plant materials to heal.

*Homeopathy:* Literally "treatment by the same." A medical system based on the principle that a substance taken in small amounts will cure the symptoms it causes when given in large amounts.

*Hydrotherapy:* The use of water for therapeutic purposes.

*Homeopathy:* The alternative tradition of administering diluted plant and mineral extracts to patients. Substances found to induce certain symptoms in a healthy person are used to counteract these symptoms in an ill person. The affect is to arouse the person's vital force and provoke healing.

*Hydrotherapy:* The ancient art of using water to promote wellness and healing.

*Imagery:* A therapeutic exercise by which the participant designs images that imagine the desired outcome. For example, the disease is seen as little black balls, a torrent of water washes the disease from the body. Some therapists provide the imagery, others counsel the client to make their own.

*Jing Hwa Chi:* A Chinese medicine and Taoist principle which means "essence transforms into energy."

*Lycopene:* Phytonutrient found in tomatoes and tomato sauce. Protects against prostate cancer and blocks UVA and UVB rays.

*Macrobiotics:* A philosophy of life, food, and health that take a wide (macro) view of life (biotics).

*Meditation:* A discipline of concentrated thought, where the breathing is controlled, and the mind is open to guidance, insight and intuition. Used for relaxation of the body as well as enlightenment of the mind.

*Melatonin:* An over-the-counter hormone that is available in health food stores. Some people use it as a sleeping aid. Others claim it has age reversing, disease fighting, and sex enhancing properties.

*Meridians:* Channels along which chi runs throughout the body.

*Mind/Body Medicine:* The idea that physical problems can be solved through conscious action of the mind.

*Muscular Strength:* Maintaining active tissue that burns calories during exercise and at rest. Done by weight and resistance training. Two thirds of muscle mass is above the hips.

*Naturopathy:* A system and a philosophy of natural healing, Naturopathy has been called "a method of curing disease by releasing inner vitality and allowing the body to heal itself."

*Neuropeptides:* Chemical messengers that control the immune system and our ability to fight disease.

*Nutraceuticals:* Natural substances found in foods that act as healing agents.

*Ojas:* Essential energy of the body that when depleted heightens susceptibility to disease.

*Orthomolecular Medicine:* A system of nutritional medicine that seeks to prevent and correct health problems by administering and varying substances that occur naturally in the human body. These are primarily vitamins, minerals, and other essential nutrients.

*Osteopathy:* A system of medical treatment that employs manipulation of the body, with special emphasis on the spine, to correct health problems.

*Phytoestrogens:* Found in soy products and alfalfa sprouts, these plant chemicals aid menopausal symptoms and may block some cancers.

*Phytonutrients:* Plant chemicals that promote health and fight disease.

*Phytosterols:* Found in plant oils, corn, sesame, soy, safflower, pumpkin, wheat, inhibit uptake of cholesterol from foods, block hormonal role in cancers.

*Polyphenols:* Protective chemicals found in apples, potatoes, plums, cherries, pears, grapes and wine, especially red wine.

*Prana:* The Ayurvedic term for energy. It is an energy of the body and the mind that is critical to the maintenance of life.

*Pranayama:* Breathing exercises used to replenish prana. Impurities are exhaled while universal energy and knowledge are inhaled.

*Progressive Relaxation:* A technique that first tenses, then relaxes muscle groups, beginning at the feet and working upwards.

*Psychoneuroimmunology:* Mind/body medicine. Therapies that employ enhanced hope, joy, and other positive emotions to enhance the effectiveness of the immune system.

*Psychooncology:* A study of behavioral techniques and therapies in the control of cancer.

*Rasayanas:* A group of herbs that promote vitality and enhance immunity.

*Resveratrol:* Protective and anti-cancer agent found in red and white grapes.

*Saponins:* Large sugarlike compounds found to have measurable pharmacological and metabolic effects on the body.

*St. John's wort:* An herb, Hypericum perforatum. *Wort* is an old English word for plant. Herbalists have said that the leaves and flowers of the plant can lighten the mood and lift the spirits. Available in health food stores.

*TCM:* Traditional Chinese Medicine. An ancient practice of natural healing which began in China and is still practiced worldwide.

*Tonic:* Foods or substances that strengthen an individual's health.

*Vijakarasana:* A group of herbs that rejuvenate the sexual organs.

*Visualization:* Also called imagery or guided imagery. A way of counseling the patient so that he or she is able to visualize in their imagination the desired outcome.

*Vitamins:* Micronutrients essential for life. Organic substances present in many foods and essential to the nutrition of humans and other animals.

*Yoga:* A discipline focusing on posture, musculature, consciousness, and breathing. The purpose of yoga is mental and physical well-being. *Yoga* is the sanskrit word for union or to join and integrate.

*Yogi:* Holy men and spiritual leaders of the Ayurvedic tradition to whom strong mental as well as physical health is attributed.

# Index

## *About the Author*

Paul Froemming is an alumnus of UCLA, with graduate degrees from Syracuse University and the University of Vermont. He has served as an education specialist with schools of medicine and nursing. His studies in natural healing have taken him to Europe, South America, and the South Pacific. He lives and writes in Santa Barbara, California.